HANDBOOK OF
Minimally Invasive
COLORECTAL SURGERY

HANDBOOK OF
Minimally Invasive
COLORECTAL SURGERY

Editors:

Nitin Mishra, MBBS, MS, MPH

Associate Professor of Surgery
Mayo Clinic Alix School of Medicine
Program Director
Department of Surgery
Mayo Clinic
Phoenix, Arizona

Abdulaziz M. Saleem, MBBS, MSc, FRCSC, FACS

Associate Professor of Surgery
Department of Surgery
King Abdulaziz University
Saudi Arabia

New York   Chicago   San Francisco   Lisbon   London   Madrid
Mexico City   New Delhi   San Juan   Seoul   Singapore   Sydney   Toronto

Handbook of Minimally Invasive Colorectal Surgery

1 2 3 4 5 6 7 8 9 DSS 28 27 26 25 24 23

ISBN 978-1-260-14285-3
MHID 1-260-14285-X

This book was set in Minion Pro by MPS Limited.
The editors were Sydney Keen Vitale and Christina M. Thomas.
The production supervisor was Richard Ruzycka.
Project management was provided by Poonam Bisht, MPS Limited.
The cover designer was W2 Design.

Library of Congress Cataloging-in-Publication Data

Names: Mishra, Nitin, editor. | Saleem, Abdulaziz M., editor.
Title: Handbook of minimally invasive colorectal surgery / editors, Nitin
    Mishra, Abdulaziz M. Saleem.
Description: New York : McGraw Hill, 2023. | Includes bibliographical
    references and index. | Summary: "A concise, step-by-step guide to
    performing minimally invasive operations in colon and rectal surgery"—
    Provided by publisher.
Identifiers: LCCN 2022031008 | ISBN 9781260142853 (paperback ; alk. paper)
    | ISBN 9781260142860 (ebook)
Subjects: MESH: Colon—surgery | Rectum—surgery | Minimally Invasive
    Surgical Procedures | Handbook
Classification: LCC RD543.C57 | NLM WI 39 |
    DDC 617.5/547—dc23/eng/20230525
LC record available at https://lccn.loc.gov/2022031008

My work in this book is dedicated to my patients, trainees, and my parents, Mr. Rajeshwar Mishra and Mrs. Indu Mishra.

—Nitin Mishra

This book is dedicated to my parents, my wife and my kids, for their continuous and unconditional love and support. In addition, this book is also dedicated to all the great surgeons that I learned from throughout my surgical training.

—Abdulaziz M. Saleem

Contents

Preface

We have written this book as a resource for surgeons who performed colorectal surgery and for trainees in colorectal and general surgery. The format of this book is such that the reader can quickly review a surgery right before performing it, we have knowingly kept the text relatively informal with an emphasis on practical tips and tricks to be used while performing an operation.

In many ways this book is meant to serve as a companion/guide for colorectal surgery faculty, fellows, and general surgery residents and should be used in conjunction with a formal textbook. The emphasis of the book is on the technical conduct of minimally invasive colorectal surgery including a brief introduction to robotic surgery. We have knowingly under played theoretical discussion of disease processes and pathology to highlight the preoperative preparation and intraoperative conduct of minimally invasive surgery. The key surgical steps have been illustrated with intraoperative pictures and diagrams for ease of comprehension and intraoperative reproduction of the illustrated techniques by the readers.

Getting Started

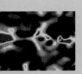

CHAPTER

1

Operating Room Setup and Patient Positioning

Supine Position

- For all right hemicolectomies, extended right hemicolectomies, and ileocolic resections, patients are placed in the supine position. The patient should be placed on either a bean bag or a gel pad to aid in securing her or him on the operating room (OR) table. Each arm should be protected by a gel pad, covering the whole length of the arm. The wrist and hand should be covered with a separate gel pad as well. The arms should be tucked in using a separate bedsheet. Make sure that the wrist is in the anatomical position, with the thumb up.

- All pressure points should be well padded.

- Check with the anesthesiologist after this step to make sure that all the intravenous (IV) lines are working. Make sure to wrap the plastic IV line lock with gauze to prevent any pressure on the skin.

- If the patient is obese, then position him or her off center on the bed, toward the ipsilateral side of the area of dissection. For example, in right hemicolectomy, place the patient on the bed off center to the right side; this is because during laparoscopy, the patient will be turned left side down, and being off center increases the safety margin if the patient were to slide. In addition, this creates space to help secure the left arm on the bed; otherwise, it might fall off the bed when the patient is tilted.

Lithotomy Position

- The lithotomy position should be the standard position for any left-sided or rectal resection, Hartmann's reversal, and any case where splenic flexure takedown is anticipated.

- The lithotomy position should be considered in certain cases of ileocolic resection for Crohn's disease, where there is an entero-sigmoid fistula. In this situation, you might need to do a sigmoid resection and use a circular stapler to establish gastrointestinal continuity. The lithotomy position will also allow access to the anus for a rigid or flexible sigmoidoscopy to leak test the repair or the anastomosis.

- The lithotomy position should be considered if the location of the lesion is not clear; or if the indication for the procedure is a small lesion, then access to the perineum is important because intraoperative colonoscopy can be used to determine the location of the lesion if it is not detected laparoscopically.

- If in doubt, one can place the patient supine, with the hip at the "break" of the table so that he or she can be placed in the lithotomy position, if needed, without having to shift the patient down.

- To place the patient in the lithotomy position, coordinate with the anesthesia team so they can control the head of the patient and the endotracheal tube.

- Make sure that there is an extra length for the IV lines prior to moving the patient. This move will require at least three people: one on either side of the bed and another holding the leg, in addition to the anesthesiologist, who is controlling the move and holding the head with the endotracheal tube.

- Move the patient down so that the buttocks sit at the edge of the bed. To assess if you are low enough, imagine that you are putting a circular stapler in the anus. Can you move it freely without the bed getting in the way? If not, then bring the patient farther down. This is to avoid having trouble while you are placing or manipulating the circular stapler.

- Place both legs in stirrups.

- The following points are important for positioning the patient:
  - Make sure that the locking clamps of the stirrups are in the same position on both sides of the bed.
  - Each knee should be in line with the patient's opposite shoulder.
  - The legs should be lower than the level of the abdomen in order to avoid hitting them as you are operating with your laparoscopic instruments through the lower abdominal ports.
  - When moving the legs out of or into the stirrups, it should be done simultaneously and slowly at the same time to avoid any injury.
  - Make sure that all the pressure points are well padded.
  - Make sure that the hips are not hyperflexed, and hyperabducted; otherwise, the inguinal ligament will compress the femoral nerve.
  - All these points should be followed to prevent knee or hip injuries, sacral pressure, and lower extremity vascular compromise. Although most of these injuries are self-limited, occasionally they will lead to prolonged disability, and this is a source of morbidity and litigation.

- The most common peripheral nerve injury is to the common peroneal nerve, by being compressed between the fibular head and the leggings or the bar holding the leg. Make sure to pad the lateral aspect of the fibula adequately to prevent nerve compression with the leggings (Figure 1-1).

⚠ Make sure that the popliteal area behind both knees is not compressed in order to prevent acute compartment syndrome.

⚠ Nerves that can be injured in this position include the following:

1. Common peroneal nerve—the most common injured nerve. Injury leads to foot drop
2. The lateral femoral cutaneous nerve
3. Femoral nerve—injured in the case of extreme thigh abduction and external rotation of the hip

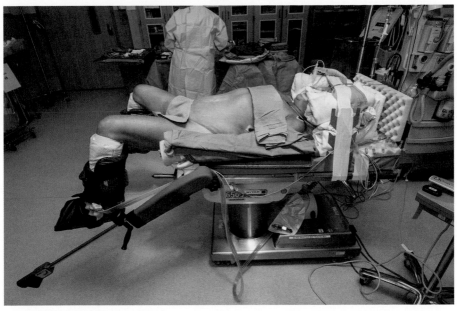

Figure 1-1. The modified lithotomy position. Note that the legs are well padded, especially laterally. In addition, notice that the head is protected on both sides and tape is placed across the head to prevent it from moving during position changes.

The Split Leg Position

- The supine split leg position has some advantages over the lithotomy position. It reduces the risk of nerve injury, compartment syndrome, the setup is easier and quicker, and it will provide access to the perineum for the stapler. Also, it will provide space for the second assistant to stand between the legs. However, this is not optimal for hand-sewn coloanal anastomosis or abdominoperineal resection as access to the perineum is limited.

Prone Jackknife Position (Figure 1-2)

- Typically, the perineal portion of the abdominoperineal resection is done with the patient in the high lithotomy position. This does not require any change in the patient position, and it will allow two teams to work at the same time if desired.

- Placing the patient in the prone position to complete the perineal portion of the abdomino-perineal resection has a number of benefits. One major advantage is that it will provide much better views for the surgeon and assistant, which make the surgery easier and are invaluable for teaching. In addition, the assistant can be helping the surgeon while he or she is standing across the table, not behind the operating surgeon, as would occur in the lithotomy position. The position of the surgeon will be more comfortable, and the ergonomics are better. In addition, the visualization of the anterior plane, which is typically the difficult part of the perineal dissection, is much better.

- However, although this approach has many advantages, it also has limitations. Changing the position of the patient in the OR to the prone jackknife position will require time and effort from all the staff, a second bed has to be available with pillows and padding to flip the patient onto the prone position (Figure 1-3). In addition, the surgeon has to finish all the dissection from the abdominal part, place the drains, mature the stoma, and close the abdomen prior to

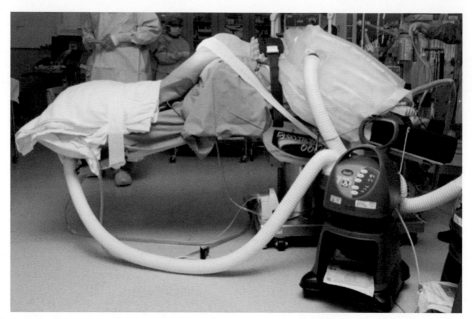

Figure 1-2. The patient is placed in the prone jackknife position. (Used with permission of Mayo Foundation for Medical Education and Research, all rights reserved.)

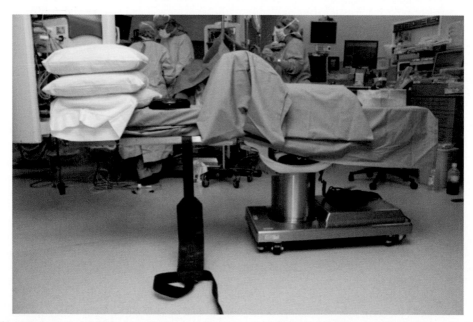

Figure 1-3. A second OR bed must be set up in the room prior to flipping a patient prone. (Used with permission of Mayo Foundation for Medical Education and Research, all rights reserved.)

flipping the patient. This will be problematic if the dissection from the abdominal part is not complete and the surgeon cannot remove the specimen or need further dissection or any kind of assistance from the abdomen. Further, it requires another OR bed to flip the patient onto, which is cumbersome if the OR room is not large enough. And understandably, this is not a favorable position for the patient from the anesthesia point of view, especially in those with a high body mass index (BMI).

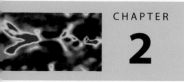

Getting the Patient Ready in the Operating Room

Background

After the patient is intubated and positioned, follow these steps to get the patient ready for surgery:

- Make sure that the operating room (OR) bed is prepared before the patient is moved to the bed (Figure 2-1).

- Place compression stockings and sequential compression devices (SCDs) on both legs, and make sure that the devices are connected and functioning.

- The patient should have a Foley catheter and orogastric tube placed as a routine in all minimally invasive cases.

- Both arms and hands should be well padded using foam or gel pads, and then both arms should be secured by tucking a bedsheet underneath the patient. Make sure that this wrap is not too tight on the arm (Figure 2-2).

- All pressure points should be well padded. Make sure that both hands are in anatomical position, with the thumbs up. After doing this, check with the anesthesiologist that the intravenous (IV) lines and oxygen saturation sensors are working. If they are not, then check for kinks or compression. The oxygen saturation probe can be moved from the fingers to the earlobes.

- The chest is taped to the OR table with 3-in. silk tape. This tape should be just below the nipple line, and the tape should be secured to the metal part on the back of the bed. Make sure that the tape is not too tight on the chest; otherwise, it might compromise the lung volume. Placing a hand under the tape while wrapping it around the patient is a simple method to avoid the wrap being too tight. After this, check with the anesthesiologist to make sure that the lung volumes are not restricted.

⚠ If the tape is placed on the chest above the nipple line, the patient might sustain neck injury if she or he slips from the bed in a reverse Trendelenburg position.

- Make sure that there is a safety strap across the thighs, without putting excessive compression on the legs.

- The anesthesiologist should secure the head so that when the bed is tilted, the head does not move (Figure 2-2).

- Add shoulder support as well. This will help to stabilize the patient during the steep Trendelenburg position. Make sure to put a gel pad between the shoulder and the shoulder support to prevent pressure injury to the shoulders.

- Place a bear hugger on top of the tape placed on the chest. Ask the anesthesiologist not to turn it on until you drape the patient; otherwise, it might touch and contaminate the prepped operative field.

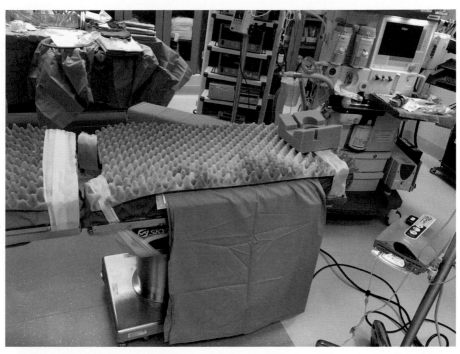

Figure 2-1. The OR bed setup, showing the gel pad, the blue bedsheet that will be used to tuck the patient's arms, and then egg crate foam on top.

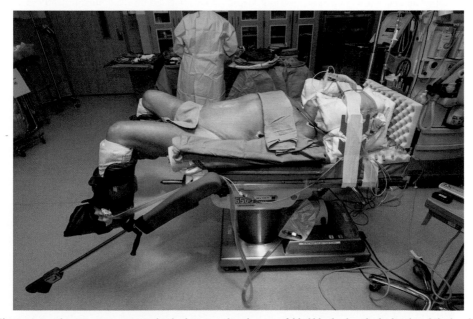

Figure 2-2. The patient is positioned in bed. Notice that there is a folded blanket beside the head, and the head is taped to prevent movement while the bed is moved in either direction. The tape (not shown) should be placed on a towel on the chest. The arms are tucked in securely. Notice the hands are covered with egg crate and positioned in the anatomical position, with the thumbs up.

- Perform the tilt test before you prep the abdomen, to make sure that the patient is well secured to the bed. Move the bed to the maximum Trendelenburg position, and then turn all the way to the right, left, and then the maximum reverse Trendelenburg position. During extreme tilting, the airway pressure and hemodynamics should be manageable from the anesthesiologist's point of view. Therefore, it's important to communicate with them to make sure that the patient will tolerate extreme position changes. Make sure that you do the tilt test gradually so that if the patient slides, you can support him or her and return the bed to the supine position.

- If the patient slides while in extreme positions despite proper taping of the chest, additional stability may be achieved by using a bean bag.

- Before you start, make sure to adjust the OR lights. For morbidly obese patients, a headlight may be useful for initial entry into the abdomen.

- Check the position of the laparoscopy towers and screens.

- For patients with an ostomy, please see chapter 10.

In summary, before you prep the patient, check the following points with the anesthesia team:

- Make sure that both IV lines are working and they are not compressed after both arms are tucked in.

- Make sure that the patient is secured on the OR table.

- Make sure that the tidal volumes are not restricted by the tape that is used to secure the patient to the table.

- Check that all the laparoscopic instruments that are needed for the operation is available in the room.

- All the instruments that are not needed immediately must be available in the room, such as open and laparoscopic staplers, various staple reloads (e.g. 2.8 mm, 3.5 mm, and 4.8 mm), the Endoloop, an energy source, and wound protectors.

- The screen and the OR lights should be appropriately positioned.

- Antibiotics are given starting 60 minutes from the beginning of the operation.

- Now you are ready for a surgical "Time-out/Pause."

Now the patient will be ready for a surgical "timeout" phase. This is performed to confirm the following facts in our institution:

- The patient's name and medical record number (MRN)

- The surgeon's name

- The diagnosis and the name of the procedure

- Site of procedure, if applicable

- Patient allergies

- The proper antibiotics, whether they were given, and what time they were given. In addition, if the antibiotics need to be redosed after a certain number of hours, then the anesthesiologist should know that.

- Whether special equipment is needed; if it is, it should be available.

- Make sure that prophylactic anticoagulation has been given as needed.

- Any other special preparation for the patient. For example, patients who are on steroids would need a stress dose.

It is important that the entire OR team pays attention during the timeout and all other activities are put on hold so that everyone listens to the person conducting the timeout, and team members can speak up if they find a discrepancy or want to bring a patient safety issue to light.

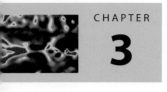

CHAPTER

3 Common Essential Steps in Laparoscopic Colorectal Surgery

Access to the Peritoneal Cavity

1. Before you start, mark the midline from the xyphoid to the pubis with a marking pen. This will help you to extend the incision in the midline if you need to do so for extraction of the specimen or conversion to an open operation.

2. A supraumbilical skin incision about 2 to 3 cm in size is made using electrocautery or a knife. If the plan is to use the midline for extraction of the specimen, then it is beneficial to make a larger skin incision (5 cm) at the very beginning of the case, especially in morbidly obese patients.

3. Use two S-retractors or Army-Navy retractors to expose the fascia. This can be done by blunt dissection using the retractors or by dividing the adipose tissue with electrocautery while the tissue is placed under tension by the retractors. The choice of method is dependent on the thickness and quality of each patient's body wall. A combination of blunt and sharp dissection works best for morbidly obese patients.

4. Use two Kocher clamps to elevate the fascia, and then divide it with scissors.

5. When you divide the fascia, limit it to the size of the port. Otherwise, it will be a source of leakage of the pneumoperitoneum, this is especially important if the initial skin incision is large, for example, you plan to extract from the midline and so have made a larger skin incision for exposure.

6. Use two Kelly clamps (or hemostats) to elevate the peritoneum—hold the peritoneum with one Kelly clamp and lift it up so that the underlying tissues are away from the clamp, hold adjacent to it with another Kelly clamp and then release the first clamp and regrasp; this is important to make sure no underlying tissue gets caught in the clamp when you take the first grasp. The peritoneum between the two clamps is then divided with a pair of scissors to gain entry into the abdomen; it is important not to make a big hole in the peritoneum because this can cause a leak in the pneumoperitoneum, a 1-cm cut is sufficient. For patients with a thicker abdominal wall, one can substitute longer instruments like a Tonsil clamp or Pean clamp. It is important not to use a perforating clamp like the Kocher clamp for this step because it can damage the underlying bowel if it is grasped in error by the surgeon.

7. To make sure that there are no adhesions before you place the port, feel the peritoneal cavity with your little or index finger or place an S-retractor in the peritoneal cavity.

8. Place two stay sutures on each side of the fascia to secure the Hasson trocar. Alternatively, use a balloon-tipped Hasson trocar.

As an alternative technique, perform the following as step number 6, that is, after dividing the fascia.

- Use your index finger or a Pean clamp and push toward the umbilicus through this fat. This will give you the quickest access.

Here are a few hints to make the procedure easier:

- In obese patients, make the skin incision longer because you will do this anyway at the end of the procedure for specimen extraction. You might as well do it from the beginning in order to achieve better exposure of the fascia and make the cutting easier. However, limit the incision on the fascia to the size of the trocar.
- Occasionally, if the patient has a long trunk or the umbilicus is not in the center, it is important to put the Hassan trocar in the center of the abdomen rather than at the level of the umbilicus. If you do not pay attention to that, and you are planning to do sigmoid resection or low anterior resection (LAR), and the camera position will be very low, your view may be compromised. An appropriate site to place the Hassan trocar would be halfway between the xiphoid and the pubis.

Position the other 5-mm ports with direct visualization via the laparoscopic camera.

⚠ Pitfall: Identify the location of the inferior epigastric vessels and avoid them while you are placing the trocars in the left or right lower quadrant.

- Inferior epigastric vessels are usually located in the area between 4 and 8 cm away from the midline.
- If you see bleeding from the inferior epigastric vessels, then perform the following actions:
  ○ If you are using a balloon-tipped trocar, inflate the balloon and pull it toward the abdominal wall to tamponade the bleeder.
  ○ If you are using a regular trocar, you can use a Foley catheter, place it through the trocar inflate the balloon, and then pull the Foley with the inflated balloon against the abdominal wall, slide the trocar out of the abdominal wall onto the proximal end of the Foley and place a hemostat on the Foley against the abdominal wall to maintain the traction in order to tamponade the bleeder. See Figure 3-1.
  ○ Next, use a suture passer to draw a figure eight around the vessel for definitive control, or alternatively, use an energy device, such as the LigaSure, to seal the bleeding vessel.
  ○ At the end of the procedure, remove all the trocars under direct supervision to ensure that there is no bleeding.

Reestablishing Pneumoperitoneum after Specimen Extraction during a Laparoscopic Procedure

Pneumoperitoneum can be reestablished in a couple of ways:

- Close the fascia in a figure eight fashion using a polydioxanone (PDS) suture and tie them except the most superior two sutures, where you can place a Hassan trocar again between them, secure the Hassan trocar using the upper two sutures, and then reestablish the pneumoperitoneum.
- Alternatively, if you are using a wound protector for specimen extraction, undo it by untwisting the top ring and then place a Hassan trocar without an obturator in the middle of the wound protector (with the balloon blown up if it is a Hasson balloon). Hold the Hassan trocar

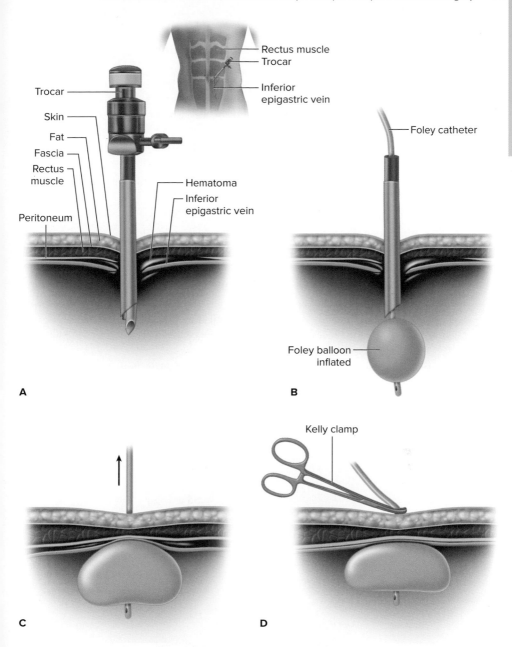

Figure 3-1. Steps illustrating the use of a balloon catheter to tamponade a bleeding inferior epigastric artery injured from insertion of a laparoscopic trocar.

and twist the wound protector around the axis of the trocar. Use an umbilical tape or 0 silk suture to tie it in place, stuff a wet lap pad between the body wall and the wound protector, and then tighten the wound protector again.

Port Sites

Port Sites for Right Hemicolectomy and Ileocolic Resection

There are a number of port configurations; however, we prefer the following:

- Three-port technique (Figure 3-2):
  - ○ Use a supraumbilical 12-mm port for the camera, and two 5-mm ports: one in the suprapubic area, and one in the LLQ.
  - ○ The LLQ port is used to retract the cecum and ascending colon during mobilization using a laparoscopic Babcock grasper, or atraumatic soft bowel grasper.
  - ○ The suprapubic port is the operating port where you can do the dissection using any energy source or monopolar laparoscopic scissors.
- Four-port technique, in a diamond configuration (Figure 3-3):
  - ○ This configuration allows you to do any colon or rectal operation.
  - ○ It also allows the assistant from the beginning of the procedure to help with retraction using the right lower quadrant (RLQ) port.
- Four-port technique, with half-crescent configuration (Figure 3-4):
  - ○ This port configuration is helpful in a formal right hemicolectomy and in cases of ileocolic resection in high body mass index (BMI) patients, where the fourth post can be used for additional retraction because the suprapubic port may not be adequate for pulling the colon during the hepatic flexure mobilization.
  - ○ The left upper quadrant (LUQ) port is helpful during the hepatic flexion mobilization, as it allows direct access to the transverse colon.
  - ○ An energy source can be used in this port while the LLQ port can be used as a retracting port during hepatic flexure mobilization.

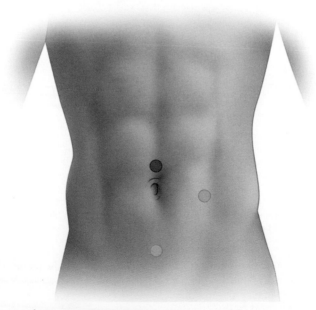

Figure 3-2. Three-port technique.

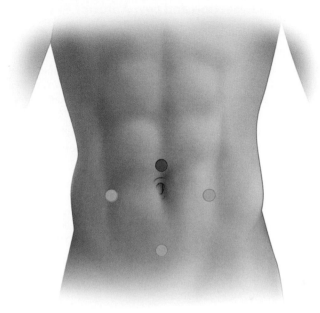

Figure 3-3. Four-port technique—diamond configuration.

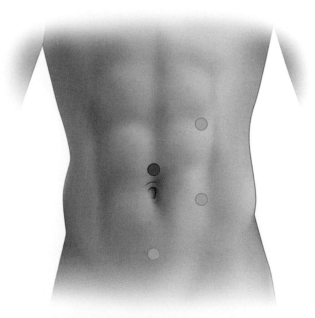

Figure 3-4. Four-port technique—half-crescent configuration.

Port Sites for Sigmoid Resection and Low Anterior Resection

- Four-port technique—diamond configuration:
  - ○ Periumbilical port (12 mm): Used for the camera.
  - ○ RLQ port (5 mm): At the beginning of the procedure, an atraumatic grasper can be utilized through this port to hold the fat at the level of the sigmoid colon and bring it medially. This port can be enlarged to 10 mm to enable the use of the Endo GIA during resection of the sigmoid colon.
  - ○ Suprapubic port: Dissecting instruments can be used through this port to mobilize the sigmoid colon and the descending colon. Laparoscopic scissors, a hook, or an energy source can be used.
  - ○ LLQ port: The initial dissection can be started with the abovementioned three ports. However, this port can be used later, during mobilization of the splenic flexure. A dissecting instrument such as a laparoscopic hook, scissors, or an energy source can be used through this port to take down the splenic flexure. To retract the colon, an atraumatic grasper can be employed through either the suprapubic port or the RLQ port. In obese patients, a long instrument may be needed if you are utilizing the suprapubic or RLQ port to retract in order to help with splenic flexure mobilization.

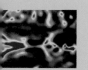

CHAPTER

4 Stoma Marking

Background

In elective cases where stoma creation is planned, patients should be seen by enterostomal nurses for ostomy marking and preoperative education. In an emergency situation, or if the stoma creation wasn't anticipated preoperatively, consider following a few simple rules.

Start by identifying the landmarks of the stoma triangle (Figure 4-1), which is formed by the umbilicus, symphysis pubis, and the anterior superior iliac spine. The patient should be examined in sitting, standing, and supine positions. Bedridden patients or patients in wheelchairs should be marked while they are in the position in which they plan to change their stoma bags.

There are many factors that should be taken into consideration to determine the best site for the stoma:

- Patient-related factors include body mass index (BMI), fat distribution (the upper abdomen has less thickness of the abdominal wall than the lower abdomen), bony prominences, skin folds, valleys, and surgical scars. The stoma location should be in the line of sight of the patient. Note that an obese patient may not be able to see the ostomy if the site of the stoma is marked below the protuberant abdomen.

- Surgical factors include stoma type (colostomy versus ileostomy) and duration (permanent versus temporary).

The stoma location should be away from any fold, bulge, valley, or bony prominence because this will cause problems with fitting stoma appliances and lead to leakage of enteric content. This is a devastating problem for patients and will affect their quality of life. In high-BMI patients, preoperative computed tomography (CT) scanning should be examined. The thickness of the abdominal wall in the upper and lower abdomen should be assessed. Typically, the lower abdominal wall is thicker than the upper abdominal wall, and hence more length is needed to bring out the ileum or the colon through the lower abdomen compared to the upper; sometimes, the length is not adequate to bring up a stoma especially if we want to Brooke it, In such situations, it is better to bring up a stoma in the upper abdomen.

The stoma should be brought through the rectus muscle to decrease the incidence of parastomal hernia. Ask the patient to lift their head from the bed, which will help you to identify the rectus muscle.

In addition, note the following points:

- The stoma site should be approximately 5 cm away from the planned midline incision.

- Make sure that it's on a flat surface to ensure adequate pouching, and that the patient can see the stoma site.

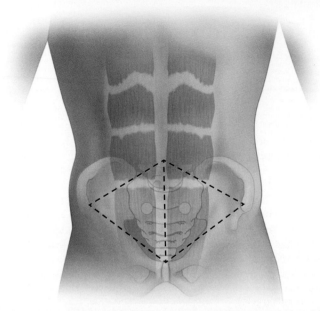

Figure 4-1. The optimal location of the stoma is through the stoma triangle, which is bounded by the umbilicus, anterior superior iliac spine, and symphysis pubis.

- The patient should be examined while lying flat, while sitting and standing. Use a marking pen to draw a mark on the site for the future stoma and cover it with 3M Tegaderm dressings. After the patient is asleep in the operating room (OR), remove the dressings and mark the stoma site before prepping the abdomen with the tip of the needle.

In cases where the creation of a permanent colostomy versus temporary ileostomy is not clear, the patient should be marked for both ileostomy and colostomy (i.e. on the right and left abdomen). In addition, in obese patients, it is preferable to mark for the stoma at two locations in each side of the abdomen; intraoperatively, the surgeon can choose which is the best site to use depending on the length of the ileum or the colon that needs to be brought up.

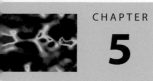

CHAPTER

5 Laparoscopic Instruments

Background

It is very important for the surgeon to be conversant with the types of laparoscopic instruments available to perform colorectal surgery. We have found it very useful to work across specialities in order to realize the entire range of instrumentation available to surgeons today, especially in bariatric surgery and gynecology. Laparoscopic instruments come in different sizes and lengths, which can be tailored to the operation in question and the patient's body habitus. The most common instruments are 5 mm in diameter and 35 to 45 cm in length. For tall and morbidly obese patients, longer bariatric instruments should be available. This chapter describes the most common instruments that are routinely available on the colorectal surgery tray for every laparoscopic operation. Of course, apart from these instruments, multiple specialized and procedure-specific instruments are available to surgeons. Figure 5-1 illustrates the instruments on a basic laparoscopic tray for colorectal surgery.

Every surgeon and surgical trainee should be familiar with the following instruments or the equivalent:

- Atraumatic graspers: In our practice, we most commonly use the atraumatic bowel grasper and the laparoscopic Babcock forceps to handle the colon, small intestine, mesentery, appendices epiploicae, omentum, and retroperitoneum. It is important to understand that the atraumatic bowel grasper tends to slip more often than the Babcock, which can be frustrating at times, but for this very reason, it tends not to tear the tissue. The Babcock has a better grasping ability but requires some operator experience regarding how much traction can be safely placed by the surgeon without tearing tissue.

- Crushing/traumatic graspers: These are important for holding fibrous or kneeling tissue such as scar or fascia, and they can also be used to hold the specimen for extraction. They typically have locking mechanisms so that tissue can be held in place without slipping, for example, Davidson and Geck (D&G) forceps.

- Needle drivers: Laparoscopic needle drivers are available in many configurations, with different gripping and release mechanism styles, and the surgeon should choose the one that works best for them.

- Monopolar scissors: Our tray typically has a 35-cm monopolar scissors with a trigger mechanism for activation. Foot-activated monopolar scissors are an alternative.

- Sealing device: We prefer the blunt-tip LigaSure device for sealing blood vessels. There are many devices available, and surgeons should choose the one with which they are most familiar and have the most experience using.

- Laparoscopic suction irrigator.

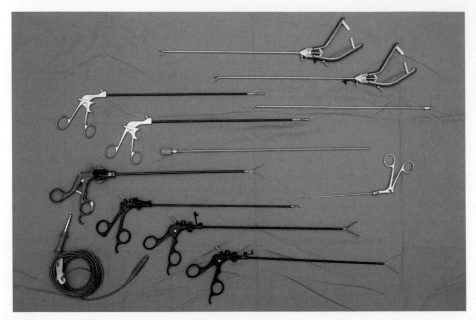

Figure 5-1. Essential instruments in a basic laparoscopic colorectal tray. Top to bottom: needle drivers × 2, D&G crushing clamp, laparoscopic needle, D&G crushing clamp, suction cannula, laparoscopic Babcock forceps, suture passer, Maryland grasper, atraumatic bowel grasper × 2, and monopolar cord.

- Laparoscopic staplers should be available as needed in varying lengths and for different tissue thicknesses.
- Maryland grasper: This is a tissue forceps that functions like the DeBakey forceps or the hemostat in an open operation (i.e. one can use it to grab a bleeding blood vessel or to hold the vascular pedicle in order to apply a clip or an ENDOLOOP). It is also very useful when closing trocar sites with suture passers and should be a component of the colorectal laparoscopic tray.
- Suture passer.
- Laparoscopic needle for doing local anesthesia blocks.
- Laparoscopic clips and ENDOLOOPS are optional, but they should be available.

Abdominal Operations

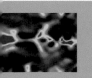

CHAPTER

6

Laparoscopic Right Hemicolectomy

Background

Right hemicolectomy involves the removal of 10 cm of the terminal ileum, cecum, ascending colon, and the proximal transverse colon. Right hemicolectomy is indicated for malignant lesions involving the right colon, including the hepatic flexure and the proximal transverse colon. In addition, it is indicated in cases of unresectable polyps, cecal diverticulitis, volvulus, and Crohn's disease. Right hemicolectomy implies division of the ileocolic, right colic, and right branch of the middle colic vessels. This can be achieved laparoscopically, laparoscopic assisted, through the open approach, or robotically.

Extended right hemicolectomy implies dividing the main trunk of the middle colic artery and extending the distal resection to include the proximal two-thirds of the transverse colon.

Preoperative Considerations

Ureteral Stents

Placement of ureteral stents should be considered in patients with:

- Severe inflammation or phlegmon involving the right lower quadrant/retroperitoneum
- A hostile abdomen
- Ureteric involvement with primary pathology demonstrated on preoperative imaging
- Morbid obesity

Intraoperative CO_2 Colonoscopy

It is prudent to have the CO_2 colonoscope in the operating room (OR) in the following situations:

- To cross-check/confirm the exact location of a lesion within the colon in the operating room.

● In ileocolic Crohn's disease where there is an ileo-sigmoid fistula. The CO_2 scope can be used to do an air leak test for the sigmoid repair/anastomosis.

Imaging

Personal review of all imaging by the surgeon is a must. In addition to the usual staging information, a surgeon should glean the following from preop scans and use them for operative planning:

● The exact location of the lesion/pathology.

● The colonic anatomy (high cecum, redundant transverse colon, prior resections, etc.).

● Involvement of adjacent organs (i.e. duodenum, ureter, sigmoid colon, and kidney). This will determine the need for supplementary procedures such as placement of ureteral stents, planning for en bloc resection of involved organs, etc.

Stoma Marking

A diverting ileostomy or creation of an end ileostomy and a mucous fistula (Prasad ostomy) should be considered in patients at a high risk for anastomotic leak, and such patients will need a preoperative stoma nurse visit and stoma marking. In a select subset of patients, one may decide to make an anastomosis and perform a proximal diverting loop ileostomy. Patients who may need diverting ileostomy after right hemicolectomy include the following:

● Patients with malnutrition—albumin <3 g/dL

● Immunocompromised patients (transplant/steroids/biologics/AIDS/uncontrolled diabetes)

● In the presence of a significant size discrepancy between the lumen of the small bowel and large bowel

● In the presence of sepsis and peritonitis

● If the patient is hemodynamically unstable, requiring persistent preoperative/intraoperative vasopressor support

Colonoscopy

If the patient has not had a colonoscopy, then a colonoscopy should be done in all patients undergoing a right hemicolectomy. This may not be possible in situations where the risk of colonoscopic perforations is prohibitive (contained perforations/inflammatory phlegmon, etc.) to rule out concomitant pathology in the rest of the colon.

Port Sites

Most cases can be done with a three-port technique. A four-port technique is preferred in obese patients, tall patients, and when proctoring a trainee.

Three-Port Configuration (Figure 6-1)

● One supraumbilical 12-mm port for the camera, and two 5-mm ports in the suprapubic area and lower left quadrant (LLQ).

● The LLQ port is used to start the medial-to-lateral dissection and ileocolic vessels division.

● The suprapubic port is the retracting port where the cecum and ascending colon is retracted in order to start the medial-to-lateral dissection.

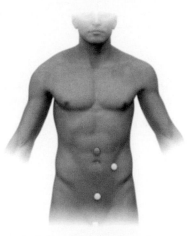

Figure 6-1. Three-port configuration for laparoscopic right hemicolectomy.

Four-Port, Diamond-Shaped Configuration (Figure 6-2)

- This configuration will allow the surgeon to do any colorectal operation.
- This will allow the assistant from the beginning of the case to help with retraction using the right lower quadrant (RLQ) port.

Four Port, Half-Crescent-Shaped Configuration (Figure 6-3)

- The left upper quadrant (LUQ) port is helpful during the hepatic flexure mobilization because it allows direct access to the transverse colon.
- An energy source can be used in the LUQ port, while the LLQ port can be used for retraction using the atraumatic grasper to continue with hepatic flexure mobilization.
- This is helpful in high body mass index (BMI) patients, and high hepatic flexure, where the dissection using the LLQ port can't reach the transverse colon.

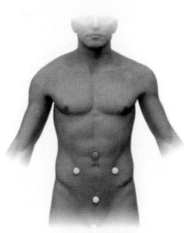

Figure 6-2. Diamond-shaped configuration for the port placement for laparoscopic right hemicolectomy.

Abdominal Operations

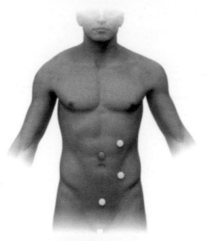

Figure 6-3. Four-port configuration (half-crescent shape).

Four-Port Configuration Plus Accessory Ports (Figure 6-4)

- This configuration can be used in cases of extended right hemicolectomy where mobilization of the distal transverse colon is needed.
- The RUQ and RLQ ports can be used to mobilize the distal transverse colon after the patient is placed in the Trendelenburg position with the left side up.

Four Approaches to Performing a Laparoscopic Right Hemicolectomy

1. Lateral-to-Medial

Advantages

- The lateral-to-medial approach is the easiest because it is similar to open surgery and the trainees will understand it better.

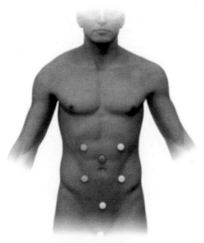

Figure 6-4. Four-port configuration plus accessory ports (accessory ports in orange colon).

- It is preferred in the following conditions:
  - ○ Thickened and foreshortened mesentery (in cases of Crohn's disease).
  - ○ Patients where it's difficult to identify the pedicle or if it is difficult to obtain adequate exposure due to excess mesenteric fat.
  - ○ Presence of mesenteric abscess or phlegmon.

Limitations

- One limitation of this approach is that the important anatomical landmarks are not identified until the end of the mobilization, such as the duodenum and the ileocolic vessels.
- Also, after the full lateral-to-medial mobilization, the colon will be very redundant and fully mobilized, and it might be difficult to take down the pedicle and do the medial dissection at that point.

Steps of the Operation

- Explore the abdominal cavity, check for ascites and carcinomatosis, and check the liver for any abnormal lesions. Make sure that the stomach is not distended, and if it is, ask the anesthetist to adjust the orogastric tube. Identify the location of the lesion. If the lesion was seen on a computed tomography (CT) scan, then most likely it can be seen intraoperatively without difficulties. The site of the lesion can show some puckering in the bowel or mass effect. Also, gentle palpation of the colon by an atraumatic grasper can provide haptic feedback on the location of the lesion because it will be firm/hard compared to the rest of the colon. Make sure that what you are feeling is not hard stool. If the gastroenterologist tattooed the area, it will make it easier to identify, especially if the tattooing was done correctly in three corners without any microperforation.
- Place the patient in a steep Trendelenburg position and turn the OR table to the left side. Rotation of the table will help move the small bowel away from the site of dissection by gravity.
- Place the omentum over the transverse colon. Reflect the small bowel out of the pelvis and away from the operation site by placing an atraumatic grasper underneath the root of the small bowel and direct it out of the pelvis (if the small bowel in the field is the terminal ileum) or upward and laterally to the left upper quadrant (if the small bowel in the field is the jejunum). Identify the important landmarks before you start, including the duodenum, cecum, and the location of the lesion in the colon.
- Mobilize the right colon: use an atraumatic grasper through the LLQ port, hold the fold of Treves to retract the colon medially (Figure 6-5). (Avoid holding the cecum, especially if the tumor is in the cecum.) Use laparoscopic scissors or an energy device through the suprapubic port with your left hand, and start by dividing the lateral attachments just medial to the white line of Toldt (Figures 6-6 and 6-7). This dissection will separate the colon and its mesentery from the retroperitoneal attachments. Once the first layer is divided, it is all right to use blunt dissection to "pull and push" the colon and the retroperitoneum to expose the correct plane of dissection. Continue with the dissection until the hepatic flexure (Figure 6-8)

🔆 **Hint:** Purple layer goes down (i.e. stays with the patient).
The color of fat of the mesocolon is dark yellow, compared to the pale yellow color of the retro peritoneum.

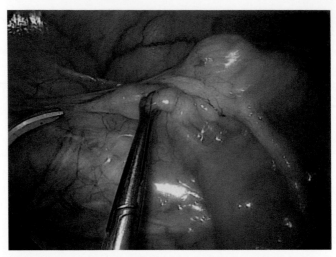

Figure 6-5. Lateral mobilization is started by holding the appendix or the fold of Treves and retract it medially. Laparoscopic scissors or LigaSure are used to start dividing the lateral attachments just medial to the white line of Toldt.

Pitfalls

⚠ Be careful when the patient is very thin, because this step may seem very easy at the beginning until you realize that the Gerota's fascia was included in the mobilization as well. The planes tend to be fused in very thin patients, patients with a lumbar hernia, or in patients with postinflammation. Stay close to the colon.

⚠ Care must be exercised during the lateral mobilization because the second portion of the duodenum may get injured. Be proactive to identify it, and then drop it down by taking down the filmy

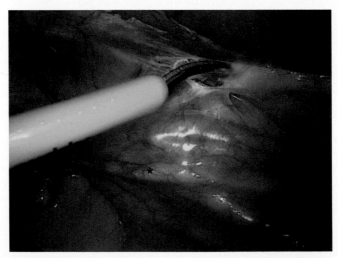

Figure 6-6. Lateral mobilization of the cecum. Notice that the right ureter (*) is crossing the right iliac artery (arrow). In thin patients, these structures can be seen without any dissection. Care must be exercised in high-BMI patients and patients who have any inflammatory process in the RLQ. Prior to starting the dissection, identify the location of the ureter, and iliac vessels, if possible. Usually, the plane of dissection is away from these structures.

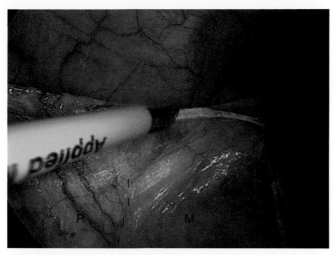

Figure 6-7. Continuing the lateral dissection just medial to the white line of Toldt. Notice the plane of dissection (dotted blue line), and notice the difference in color between the mesentery of the colon, which is dark yellow (M), and the pale yellow in the retroperitoneum (R).

attachments between duodenum and right mesocolon and gently sweeping down the duodenum. Be mindful when you do this step and avoid using an energy source. This can be done bluntly or sharply but without the use of energy (Figures 6-9 and 6-10).

- Hepatic flexure mobilization: Adjust the bed now to the reverse Trendelenburg position. Use an energy source through the LLQ port, divide the hepatic flexure attachments while using an atraumatic grasper through the suprapubic port to retract the transverse colon caudally (Figure 6-11).

- Adding an LUQ port will make this step easier (Figure 6-3), especially in high-BMI patients. In that situation, use an energy source through the LUQ port to divide the hepatic flexure attachment, while using the LLQ port for retraction. If still there are difficulties or there is

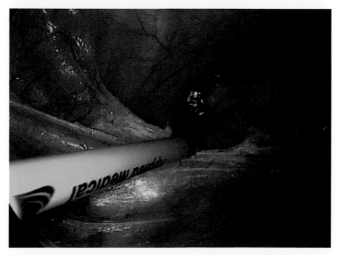

Figure 6-8. The lateral dissection is continued until the hepatic flexure is reached.

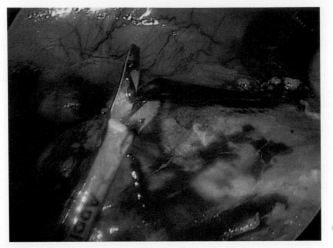

Figure 6-9. After taking down the hepatic flexure attachments, be mindful of the duodenum (*) and continue with taking these hepatic flexure attachments close to the colon as safely as possible.

a need for the assistant to retract the colon to get a better exposure, place a port in the RLQ because this will help with retraction. In addition, the assistant can use the suprapubic port for retraction.

- Decide if you are taking the omentum with the colon or leaving it. Consider taking the omentum in cases of tumors involving the transverse colon or if the tumor is at the hepatic flexure.
- If you decide to resect part of the omentum, then reflect the omentum inferiorly. Identify where the transverse colon is in relation to the stomach. Start dividing the omentum in between and enter the lesser sac. There is an area in the omentum that is transparent and you can start dissection from that area to get into the lesser sac (Figure 6-12). Continue with this dissection until you reach the hepatic flexure. Make sure that you are away from the gallbladder, stomach,

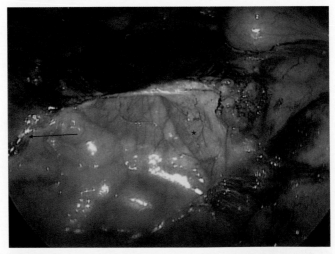

Figure 6-10. After the hepatic flexure is taken down (arrow), notice the duodenum (*) is now clear. Be mindful during the initial mobilization of the flexure about the location of the duodenum to avoid any injury.

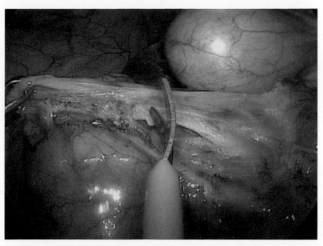

Figure 6-11. Taking down the hepatic flexure attachments, after pulling the hepatic flexure caudally and upward to better expose the attachments.

and the duodenum at all times. You can show yourself the path of dissection by using an atraumatic grasper to do gentle blunt dissection toward the hepatic flexure, and this will guide you to where the dissection should be and make the operation safer by minimizing the chance of injuring the colon, duodenum, or gallbladder.

- Identify the middle colic vessels. There are two ways to identify them. It's not always easy especially if the mesentery is thick due to a high BMI. If the vessels are easily identified, you can divide them intracorporeally, which will make the extraction easier.

  ○ The first approach is from the top. Pull the transverse colon at the hepatic flexure caudad and toward the abdominal wall. This will put the middle colic vessels on stretch and make them easy to identify. Divide the middle colic vessels using an energy source.

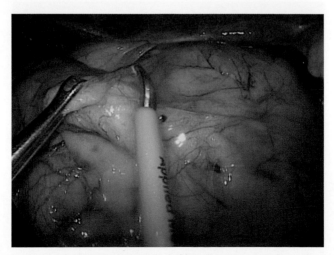

Figure 6-12. Starting the hepatic flexure takedown by holding the transverse colon with an atraumatic grasper and pulling it caudally, and start in between the stomach (*) and the transverse colon.

Pitfalls

⚠ When you do this step, make sure that you relax on your retraction with your left hand; otherwise, once you start dividing the vessel, if you are applying excessive tension, the vessel will tear and retract and cause major bleeding. Relax the retraction slightly and apply the energy source as proximal as you need on the vessel in two different locations close to each other, and then more distally (toward the specimen side) and then divide in between.

- The second method is from inferiorly, where you reflect the omentum superiorly above the transverse colon and then left up the transverse colon at the hepatic flexure cranially and upward toward the abdominal wall. This will put the middle colic vessels on stretch and make them easy to identify. Divide it using an energy source.

- This step is optional, and you can do it extracorporeally. However, be mindful when you extract the specimen not to apply excessive traction; otherwise, the middle colic vessels may tear and cause major bleeding. Be mindful that if the ligation of the middle colic vessels is done extracorporeally, the incision can be extended cranially to allow for better visualization when performing this step.

- Assess how well the colon is mobilized, and check if you need to do further mobilization. If the colon can be rolled medially beyond the midline and you can see the "C" of the duodenum, then it's mobilized enough for extraction.

- The terminal ileum should be mobilized as well by dividing its attachments off the retroperitoneum.

- In the case of extended right hemicolectomy, you can insert two additional ports, one in the RUQ and one in the RLQ, to help with mobilizing the distal transverse colon and splenic flexure, if needed (Figure 6-4).

Pitfalls

⚠ During mobilizing the terminal ileum, be mindful that If you are too lateral or too deep, you risk injuring the right iliac vessels (Figure 6-13) and the right ureter, and if you are too medial, then you

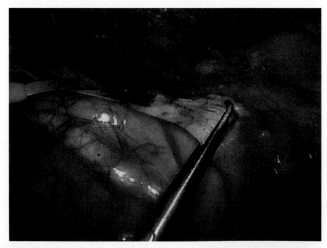

Figure 6-13. Mobilization of the lateral attachments that is holding the terminal ileum after the right colon is mobilized. Note that the right iliac artery (*) is close by and the dissection should be away and close to the cecum as safely possible.

may cause bleeding from the mesentery of the small bowel. It is imperative to be in the correct plane—this plane can be identified by grasping the terminal ileum and retracting it toward the abdominal wall and then back to its physiological position several times, while paying attention to the layer that slides over the retroperitoneum when this is done. This is the layer that should be divided to get into the correct plane.

Use minimal or no cautery and try to dissect gently and sweep in the appropriate planes.

- Place a laparoscopic locking grasper on the fold of Treves. Make sure that the colon and small bowel are in their anatomical location, to avoid twisting of the small bowel or colon during extraction.

- Extend the incision cephalad and caudad, but keep the incision small, and if the specimen can't be extracted from that incision, then extend it 1 cm at a time until the specimen is out.

- Consider extending the incision preferentially in the following ways:

  ○ Caudad, if you are doing an ileocolic resection for Crohn's disease, where you would not need to exteriorize the transverse colon and omentum. In addition, it will help to exteriorize the diseased terminal ileum.

  ○ Cephalad, if you are doing a formal right hemicolectomy for cancer, to make it easier to extract the transverse colon (and omentum) and to do the ileo-transverse anastomosis. Also, if the middle colic vessels are not divided intracorporeally.

- Place your index finger on the umbilicus and go around it to make the incision close to the midline as possible and to help you make it symmetrical. Go to the left of the umbilicus in cases where you might anticipate making a right-sided ileostomy.

- Place a wound protector and then extract the colon. Before you fold the wound protector on itself, place your index finger inside the abdominal cavity along the abdominal wall, and sweep inside around the abdominal part of the wound protector, to make sure that nothing is caught underneath it.

Causes of Difficulty with Extracting the Specimen

1. Small skin/fascial incision. In this case, place your finger inside the abdominal cavity and sweep around, and see where the specimen is mainly stuck, and then extend the fascia and skin either cranially or caudally accordingly. This can be done while the specimen in the wound. Basically, use a retractor, like Langenbeck, and retract the skin, and place a finger underneath the fascia to protect the bowel underneath and then divide the fascia using electrocautery.

2. Suction effect. Use your finger and sweep around the colon to break any suction effect, and then try to pull the colon with back-and-forth motions. Make sure that you don't rotate the colon while doing this move, and pull it straight up.

3. If you do not divide the middle colic vessels intracorporeally, it may tether the colon and make extraction challenging. Excessive traction during extraction can tear these vessels and cause major bleeding. Typically, a gush of bleeding will be evident. Rarely, the anesthesiologist will alert you about hypotension with no apparent bleeding because a bulky colon being extracted through a small incision may obscure your view.

   If in doubt as to why extraction is challenging, one can always reestablish the pneumoperitoneum and look inside the abdomen as to what the problem is, it is safer to look and resolve the issue laparoscopically than extracorporeally.

- After the colon is exteriorized, assess the location of the lesion. Then identify the proximal and distal resection margin. If the surgery is for cancer, make sure to include the last 10 cm of the terminal ileum (TI) with the resection specimen.

Abdominal Operations

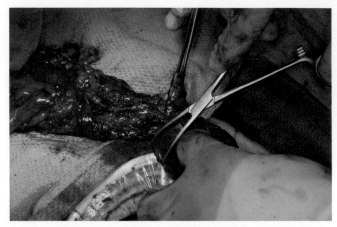

Figure 6-14. Clearing the small bowel from mesentery in preparation for creating the anastomosis.

- Divide the TI and the transverse colon using a GIA stapler with a 3.5-mm staple height. In a very thickened small bowel due to Crohn's disease, you may consider using a 4.8-mm staple height (rarely needed). Make sure that the stapler is angled toward the antimesenteric border of the ileum.

- Divide the transverse colon using the GIA stapler with a 3.5-mm staple height with the antimesenteric tenia of the colon being at the corner of the stapler. In case of Crohn's disease, divide at the level of the ascending colon.

- Divide any remaining mesentery/mesocolon with clamps and ties or an energy device (Figure 6-14).

- Open the specimen to confirm the resection of pathology before sending it to the pathologist. If happy with the specimen and margins, then proceed to make the anastomosis.

Anastomosis

- Side-to-side functional end-to-end anastomosis is performed.

- Make sure that the orientation of the small bowel and the colon are correct and there is no twist in the mesentery. Slide your index finger along the small bowel mesentery to make sure there is no twist—the mesenteric edge should be straight.

- Align the small bowel and transverse colon and place three stay sutures using 3-0 silk stitches. Place these seromuscular bites in the bowel very close to the mesenteric edge. This will isolate the mesentery when you perform the anastomosis. This step is optional.

- Place a blue towel underneath the wound protector so you can put all the "dirty" instruments on it.

- Divide the antimesenteric corner of the small bowel and large bowel using curved Mayo scissors or electrocautery.

- Lift the mucosa where you already made the cut, and divide it again, confirm that you are in the lumen and that the size of the hole is adequate to allow insertion of the stapler without difficulty.

- Insert the thin part of the stapler in the small bowel, and the other part in the colon.

- While you are inserting the stapler, make sure you are watching the tip of the stapler because it might injure the bowel wall.

- Align both halves of the stapler and close it.
- Make sure that you are able to sweep your finger behind the stapler to confirm that there is no mesentery incorporated in the stapler. This step is not necessary if you place the stay sutures described above.
- Fire the stapler in a controlled fashion.
- When you open the stapler, it should be done in a controlled fashion to avoid stretching the anastomosis.
- Use a ring forceps to open the lumen of the bowel to inspect the staple line and make sure there is no active bleeding. If there is, you can use 3-0 silk and oversew the bleeder.
- Offset the staple line to prevent the two staple lines becoming stuck to each other because this may lead to postoperative obstruction.
- Close the common enterotomy—colotomy with Allis clamps. Make sure in this step to take small bites but you should include the full thickness of the bowel on both sides. Start from the middle, followed by the corners, and then in between.
- Closure of the enterotomy–colotomy defect either with another firing of the GIA stapler, TA stapler, or hand sewn. Prior to firing the stapler to close the common enterotomy–colotomy defect, make sure that after you place the stapler, there is a patent anastomosis and it's not shorted or narrowed after placing the GIA stapler to close the defect. Be mindful of that.
- Place two crotch stitches at the bifurcation of the two limbs of bowel where the liner stapler ends. This will decrease the tension on the staple line.
- Omentoplasty: If possible, then the omentum should be draped over the anastomosis and secured by a stitch.

Another technique used to perform this anastomosis is the Barcelona technique.

Advantages of the Barcelona Technique

- It saves two staple loads.
- The risk of twisting the bowel, either the colon or small bowel, is minimal.
- Technique: (Figures 6-15 to 6-25)
  - Exteriorize the colon and the terminal ileum.
  - Identify the proximal and distal resection margins.
  - Clear the small bowel, and large bowel mesentery at the level of resection.
  - Make an enterotomy and colotomy on the specimen side of the bowel.
  - Perform the side-to-side, functionally end-to-end anastomosis using the GIA stapler blue load, as described previously.
  - Then use another firing of the GIA stapler to close the common defect.
- Place two crotch stitches at the bifurcation of the two limbs of bowel where the liner stapler ends. This will decrease the tension on the staple line.
- Omentoplasty: If possible, then the omentum should be draped over the anastomosis and secured by a stitch.
- After anastomosis is completed, return the bowel to the abdomen. Remove the blue towel with all the dirty instruments used during the anastomosis and remove it from the operative field. The surgical team should change gloves.

Abdominal Operations

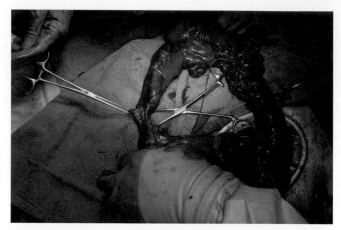

Figure 6-15. Creating an enterotomy and colotomy after the mesentery is cleared at that level in the terminal ileum and transverse colon.

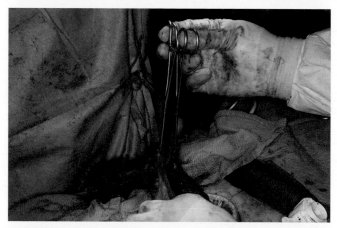

Figure 6-16. Aligning the terminal ileum and transverse colon after the enterotomy and colotomy were made.

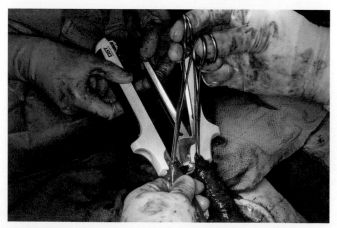

Figure 6-17. Inserting the GIA stapler in the terminal ileum and transverse colon.

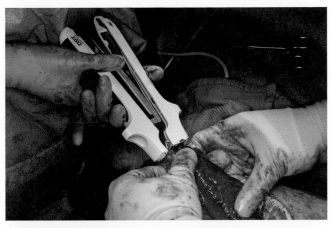

Figure 6-18. Closing the GIA stapler.

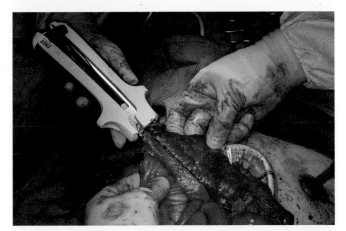

Figure 6-19. The assistant is making sure that the mesentery of the terminal ileum and transverse colon are not caught in the stapler, by placing both hands underneath the bowel and pulling the mesentery away from the stapler.

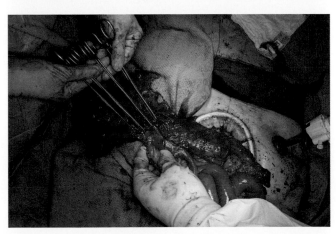

Figure 6-20. After the side-to-side functionally end-to-end anastomosis is created, then the common enterotomy–colotomy defect is closed with multiple Allis clamps.

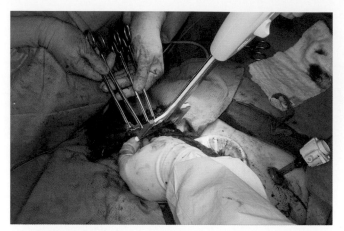

Figure 6-21. A TA stapler is placed across the common enterotomy–colotomy defect, just underneath the Allis clamps.

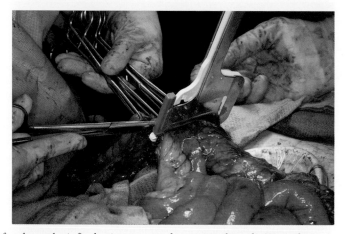

Figure 6-22. After the stapler is fired, scissors are used to cut just above the TA stapler.

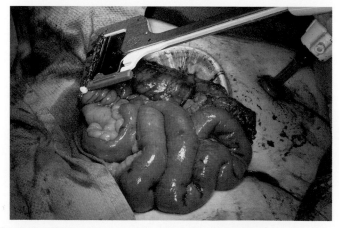

Figure 6-23. After the bowel is cut (specimen), then the TA stapler is opened.

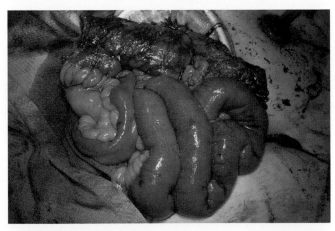

Figure 6-24. The ileocolic anastomosis.

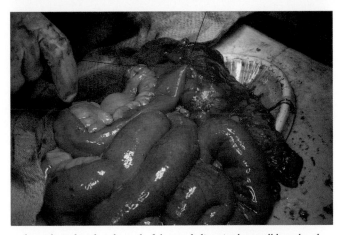

Figure 6-25. A crotch stitch is placed at the end of the staple lines in the small bowel and transverse colon.

- You now have two options:
  - ○ First option: retract the abdominal wall at the extraction site with an Army-Navy retractor and use the laparoscopic light held with a large Babcock forceps to see the trocars from inside the abdominal cavity and remove them under direct vision. Inspect the abdomen for hemostasis and close the fascial and skin incisions. This approach is useful in thin patients.
  - ○ Second option: reestablish pneumoperitoneum. Check laparoscopically for hemostasis. Make sure again that there is no twist in the mesentery of the small bowel. Remove ports under direct vision. All the fascial defects > = 10 mm should be closed. A suture passer can be used for closure, especially in obese patients.

There are several ways to reestablish pneumoperitoneum

- Close the fascia of the extraction site and use a 5-mm camera through the other ports to visualize. In this method, the last port comes out without internal visualization (typically the suprapubic which has the least likelihood of causing major bleeding). The disadvantage of doing this is depending on 5-mm camera to visualize, which may not be the best option. In addition, it will leave the surgeon with one working port, which is the suprapubic port.

- Close the fascia of the extraction site in a figure-of-eight fashion and tie them except the two cephalad sutures, where one can place the Hasson trocar in-between, secure the Hasson trocar using the upper two sutures, and then reestablish pneumoperitoneum.

- Or, if using a wound protector, undo it, and then place the Hasson trocar without an obturator in the middle of the wound protector (blow up the balloon if it's a balloon Hasson) and hold the Hasson trocar and twist the wound protector around the axis of the Hasson trocar. Tie an umbilical tape, or 0-silk suture around it and then place a wet lap around the wound protector and twist the ring of the wound protector again.

2. Medial-to-Lateral

- Dividing the pedicle intracorporeally will facilitate high ligation of the ileocolic pedicle, especially in high-BMI patients where this step would be difficult if it was done extracorporeally. Also, doing this intracorporeally will decrease the length of the incision for extraction.

- Preferred in cancer cases.

Advantages

- The advantage of this approach is that the important landmarks in this operation are identified at the beginning of the case, such as the ileocolic vessels, and the duodenum.

- In addition, the colon will be still attached laterally (white line of Toldt) and thus the colon will be naturally suspended and will not fall into the view and allow for medial to lateral dissection. So keeping the lateral dissection later will help to "self" retract the colon from the lateral part to facilitate the medial dissection.

- Minimal manipulation of the tumor (no touch technique).

Limitations

- This approach is not the usual approach during open surgery, and thus it will require practice and training to be familiar with the planes.

Steps of the Operation

- Patient setup is the same as the lateral-to-medial technique.

- Consider using the diamond ports configuration because the RLQ port will be helpful to expose the pedicle by the assistant.

- After you reflect the omentum over the transverse colon, and sweep the small bowel away, identify the duodenum. The duodenum can be easily identified without any need for dissection in thin patients.

- During this approach, be mindful that the duodenum is very close and at risk for injury.

- The assistant can use the RLQ port to stretch the ileocolic pedicle by grasping the mesentery of the colon just medial to the cecum and pull it gently laterally and toward the abdominal wall (Figure 6-26). However, in three-port configuration, the surgeon can hold the cecum with their left hand using the suprapubic port, and start the dissection using the LLQ port.

- Use hook, scissors, or LigaSure to score just underneath and parallel to the stretched ileocolic vessels. Typically, there is a "valley" in this location. (Figures 6-27 to 6-29)

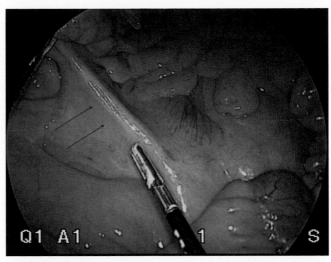

Figure 6-26. After reflecting the omentum above the transverse colon, and sweeping the small bowel away, the ileocolic pedicle (arrows) is put on stretch by holding the fat close to the cecum and pulling it laterally and toward the ceiling. Notice the duodenum in this view (star).

- Use an atraumatic grasper in the suprapubic port to lift up the ileocolic pedicle gently, while using a LigaSure or an atraumatic grasper to do the dissection bluntly. The dissection should dissect the mesentry of the right colon off the retroperitoneum. The move of the right hand should be from 12 o'clock to 6 o'clock in a straight line (Figure 6-30).
- Once the medial-to-lateral dissection has started, the duodenum will be seen medially (Figure 6-31). Divide the filmy attachments on top of the duodenum to drop the duodenum down completely (Figure 6-32).

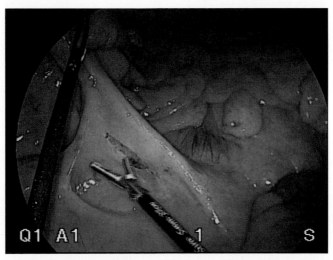

Figure 6-27. Starting the dissection by creating a window underneath the ileocolic vessels with the LigaSure by dividing only the peritoneal layer. Alternatively, laparoscopic scissors are used to score underneath the vessel.

Abdominal Operations

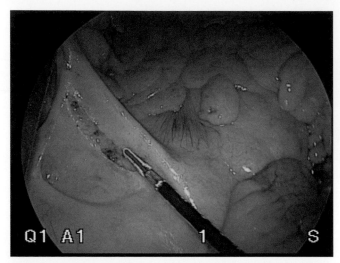

Figure 6-28. Extend this window along the ileocolic vessels to facilitate the medial-to-lateral dissection.

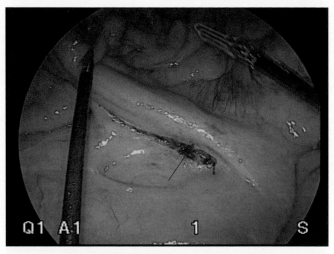

Figure 6-29. After the peritoneal layer underneath the ileocolic vessel is scored, the medial-to-lateral dissection should start. Again, notice the duodenum very close to the origin of the ileocolic vessels.

- Do not use electrocautery while dissecting near the duodenum to avoid any thermal injury. If you are using the LigaSure, use the cut only to divide these transparent and filmy attachments to drop the duodenum completely down (Figure 6-33).

- Continue with the dissection until you reach the hepatic flexure from this dissection.

- The medial dissection is completed when the surgeon reaches the transverse colon superiorly, the white line of Toldt laterally, and duodenum medially. The dissection should not extend medial to the duodenum, because of risk of vascular injury (Figures 6-34 to 6-36).

- After that is done, the next step is to divide the ileocolic vessel. The ileocolic vessels should be grasped with an atraumatic grasper, and with the LigaSure or another atraumatic grasper.

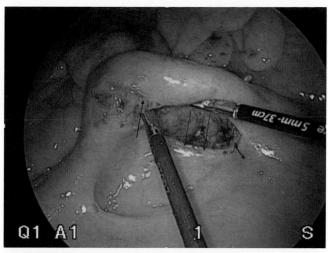

Figure 6-30. Medial-to-lateral dissection started by placing an atraumatic grasper with the left hand directed upward (blue arrow) and with the right hand, the LigaSure or, alternatively, an atraumatic grasper, to do the dissection. The direction of the dissection should be from 12 o'clock to 6 o'clock (red arrows).

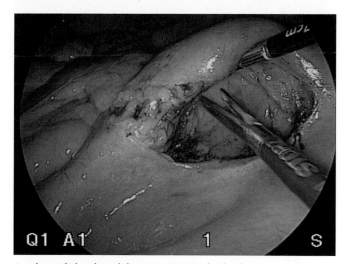

Figure 6-31. Starting the medial-to-lateral dissection. Notice the duodenum is nearby.

A window is created from the other side of the ileocolic vessels. Always superiorly there is a bare area that can be dissected in order to isolate the ileocolic pedicle for ligation. The peritoneum over the ileocolic vessel should be scored or thinned, especially if the mesentery is bulky (Figures 6-36 to 6-39).

- After the division of the ileocolic vessels, divide the lateral attachments of the right colon by grasping the fold of Treves and pulling it medially and upward. There should be minimal attachments at that point, and any that remain can be taken easily.

Abdominal Operations

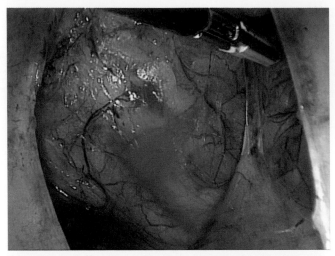

Figure 6-32. Medial dissection, where the duodenal attachments are divided to drop down the duodenum.

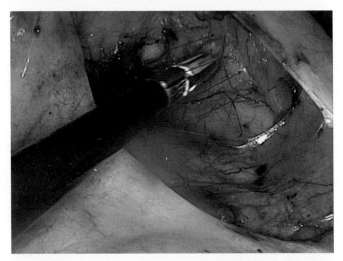

Figure 6-33. Medial dissection. Notice the area of dissection, which is the line that separates the retroperitoneum from the mesentery of the colon. The color of the fat is different.

- Now, you can start from the transverse colon and follow the steps as discussed in the lateral-to-medial approach.

Hint: If it's difficult to start the medial-to-lateral dissection, due to, for example, the small bowel being stuck to the pedicle, you can do the medial-to-lateral dissection by scoring the peritoneum in the "valley" above the ileocolic pedicle (rather than below it). In such situations, it is wise to combine medial-to-lateral and lateral-to-medial approaches to avoid injury to the duodenum.

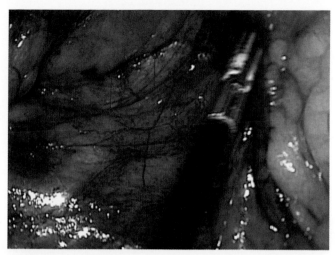

Figure 6-34. After completing the division of the ileocolic pedicle, further dissection is carried out toward the transverse colon. Notice the red arrows indicating the line of separation and the area of dissection. Notice the duodenum (star) is close to the area of dissection.

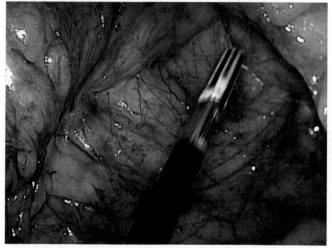

Figure 6-35. Further dissection is carried out laterally toward the white line of Toldt. The arrows show the area of dissection.

3. Top-Down

The top-down approach can be useful when there is a large phlegmon in the RLQ and it is difficult to appreciate the plane around the cecum. Thus, one can start from the hepatic flexure, find a virgin plane, and then go down toward the pathology.

Advantages

- This approach is very useful when there is a large tumor in the ascending colon or cecum and the right colon is hard to mobilize due to tumor size.

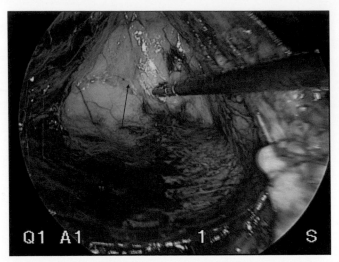

Figure 6-36. Continue with medial-to-lateral dissection until the transverse colon (blue arrow) is reached from the medial approach.

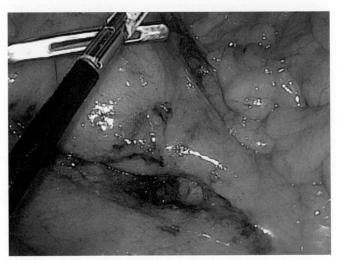

Figure 6-37. After the medial dissection is complete, then the ileocolic pedicle is grasped and stretched out in preparation for division.

- This approach is also useful for complicated Crohn's disease (with phlegmon, abscess, or enterocutaneous fistula) involving the terminal ileum.
- In these situations, start the mobilization from the top down, away from the tumor or phlegmon, and start at the hepatic flexure. This would allow the operator to start the mobilization from a normal plane in the hepatic flexure and then direct the dissection toward the correct plane along the ascending colon.

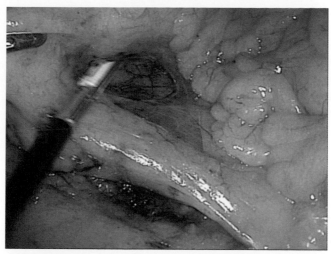

Figure 6-38. There is almost always a clear window cephalad to the ileocolic vessels that need to be cleared prior to dividing the ileocolic vessels.

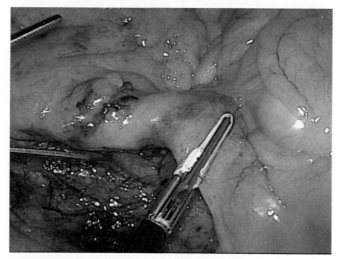

Figure 6-39. Division of the ileocolic pedicle. Care must be taken to check on the duodenum and make sure that it's not injured during ligation of the pedicle.

Limitations

- This is not the most common approach, and starting at the hepatic flexure may be challenging in patients with bulky omentum and those who have had prior gall bladder or liver surgery.

Steps of the Operation

- Start by mobilizing the hepatic flexure. Place the bed in the reverse Trendelenburg position and tilt the table to the left.

Abdominal Operations

- Use the suprapubic port to hold the hepatic flexure gently caudad, and then with the port in the LLQ, use the LigaSure to start the dissection.
- Prior to starting the dissection, identify the location of the gallbladder, hepatic flexure, and stomach in relation to the site of the dissection.
- Be mindful not to injure the gallbladder by excessive retraction with the left hand.
- Start taking the hepatic flexure layer by layer, until the flexure is taken down. After that, continue to mobilize the ascending colon until the cecum is reached.
- In case of Crohn's disease, the difficult part would be mobilization of the cecum. However, establishing a normal plain starting from the hepatic flexure downward will facilitate the identification of the normal plane in the cecum.

4. Inferior-to-Superior

This approach can be used if the usual medial-to-lateral approach is difficult due to thick mesentery caused by Crohn's disease, obesity, or prior surgery. Also, it can be used if the lateral-to-medial approach is difficult.

Advantages

- Identifying the critical structures at the beginning of the case, including the right ureter, right iliac vessels, and the duodenum, before the dissection is started.
- It might be an easier approach in Crohn's disease or redo operations.

Limitations

- Mobilization of the duodenum unintentionally.
- Higher likelihood of Injuring the duodenum or the inferior vena cava.

Steps of the Operation

- Sweep the small bowel out of the pelvis.
- Identify the terminal ileum.
- Identify the critical structures in this approach, the right ureter and right iliac artery.
- Lift up the mesentery of the terminal ileum and then incise the peritoneum with laparoscopic scissors or hook just above and parallel to the right iliac artery and right ureter.
- After lifting up the mesentery of the terminal ileum, create the plane between the retroperitoneum and mesentery of the right colon using atraumatic grasper.
- Take down the attachments to drop down the duodenum. Avoid the dissection medial to the duodenum.
- After reaching the hepatic flexure from the medial dissection, the next step is to divide the ileocolic vessels as described in the medial-to-lateral approach.

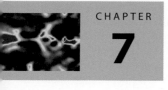

Laparoscopic Ileocolic Resection for Crohn's Disease

Background

Ileocolic resection involves removal of the terminal ileum, and the cecum. This is not an oncological resection, and it is indicated for benign conditions such as Crohn's disease of the terminal ileum. One of the major technical differences from a formal right hemicolectomy for cancer is that the right branch of the middle colic artery is not divided and the ileocolic pedicle is not divided close to its origin. In addition, the resection of the cecum/ascending colon is limited, because in most cases, the rest of the colon is normal. However, despite this fact, most cases require hepatic flexure mobilization in order to extract the colon from a midline incision in order to perform an extracorporeal anastomosis.

Preoperative Considerations

Ureteral Stents

In most right-sided colon resections, ureteral stents are not needed; however, in cases where there is an inflammatory process in the right lower quadrant (RLQ) that is close to the ureters on preoperative imaging or is distorting the normal anatomy, it is prudent to use stents. Placing a ureteral stent will help identify the ureter intraoperatively and, if injury should happen, it will likely be recognized and repaired.

Complete Evaluation of the Small Bowel

All patients with Crohn's disease should have a recent evaluation of the small bowel by either computed tomography enterography or magnetic resonance enterography. The following important information can be obtained from preoperative imaging that will help to plan the surgical intervention:

- The location of the pathology.
- Type of the disease, either fistulizing or stricturing in nature.
- The length of the diseased segment.
- Presence of any fistula or any communication to other structures. If there is a fistula, then determine if the other structure is diseased (e.g. in the case of an ileo-sigmoid fistula).
- Determining if there are any skips lesions, their location, and their distance from the index lesion.

Endoscopy

Full evaluation of the gastrointestinal tract is essential prior to surgery. Upper and lower endoscopy is needed to assess the disease distribution prior to surgery. Colonoscopy will show if there is any colonic involvement. In addition, in cases of ileo-sigmoid fistula, it will determine if the sigmoid colon is the primary site of Crohn's colitis or is secondarily affected by the inflamed terminal ileum. This would help to manage this intraoperatively, in the former scenario, the patient might require formal sigmoid resection, whereas in the latter, a primary repair of the sigmoid colon will be sufficient. In addition, the preoperative colonoscopy is important to document that there is no disease in the right colon, where the anastomosis will take place. Demonstration of the lack of inflammation in the colon left behind after the surgery is important, especially in patients who get a diverting ileostomy at the time of surgery. It helps in differentiating between diversion colitis and Crohn's disease in the postoperative period prior to reversal of the ileostomy.

Medications

Patients with Crohn's disease may be on medications with different side effect profiles, such as anti-TNF, immunomodulators, and steroids. Detailed medication history is important, because it might affect the type and timing of the procedure performed.

Biologics

In elective settings, we recommend stopping anti-TNF medications 3–4 weeks prior to surgery. In emergency situations, if the patient is on an anti-TNF agent, then creation of a stoma should be strongly considered, with or without an ileocolic anastomosis.

Steroids

Patients who are taking steroids (more than 5 mg of prednisone) for 3 weeks or longer should be considered a candidate for stress dose of steroids, we use hydrocortisone 50 to 100 mg IV in the perioperative area before surgery. Patients who are on greater than 10 mg per day dose of prednisone are considered to be at a higher risk for anastomotic leak.

Stoma Marking

A diverting ileostomy or creation of end ileostomy and mucous fistula (Prasad) should be considered in patients at high risk for anastomotic leak and these patients will need a preoperative stoma nurse visit and stoma marking. Patients who may need intestinal diversion in cases of Crohn's disease include:

- Severe malnutrition—albumin <3 g/dL.
- Septic patient.
- Immunocompromised patients (steroids/biologics/uncontrolled diabetes/AIDS/posttransplant immunosuppression).
- Poor tissue quality noted during surgery.
- Gross discrepancy in the caliber and thickness of the ileum and colon due to chronic disease.

Positioning

In a standard laparoscopic right hemicolectomy, the supine position with both arms tucked in is the usual position we follow in these cases. This applies to most cases of Crohn's disease. However, in the case of a Crohn's disease patient with a fistula between the small bowel and the sigmoid colon (ileosigmoid fistula), consider placing the patient in the lithotomy position. In these cases, one may need to perform an intraoperative CO_2 flexible sigmoidoscopy and there might be a need of doing a sigmoid resection if the sigmoid colon is diseased. A flexible sigmoidoscopy may help delineate extent of disease and to perform an air leak test if a primary repair or resection of the sigmoid colon is carried out.

Steps of the Operation

In cases of Crohn's disease, the lateral-to-medial approach is preferable because the mesentery is thickened and foreshortened.

Both the surgeon and the assistant stand on the patient's left side with the monitor located across the patient, facing them.

Mobilization of the Colon and Terminal Ileum: Lateral-to-Medial and Inferior-to-Superior Approach

- Start by placing the patient in the Trendelenburg position with the right side up. Reflect the greater omentum above the transverse colon. Assess the RLQ and assess the cecum and the terminal ileum. Identify the diseased segment. If any segment of disease is identified in the small intestine with preoperative imaging, then it should be identified at this point of the operation (Figures 7-1 and 7-2).

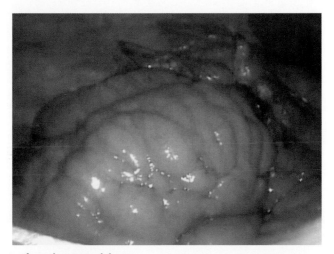

Figure 7-1. Creeping fat in the terminal ileum.

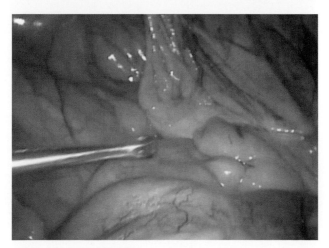

Figure 7-2. Identification of the terminal ileum.

Abdominal Operations

- Start by holding the appendix with an atraumatic grasper through the lower left quadrant (LLQ) port and direct it medially and toward the abdominal wall. With the left hand, use laparoscopic scissors connected to electrocautery or any vessel-sealing device through the suprapubic port and divide the lateral attachments (Figures 7-3 to 7-6).

- Mobilize the cecum and the ascending colon from the retroperitoneal structures. The terminal ileum is identified and mobilized as well, taking great care not to injure the right ureter or gonadal vein (Figures 7-7 to 7-9).

⚠ Pitfalls: Great care should be exercised while completing the lateral-to-medial mobilization to avoid the duodenal injury.

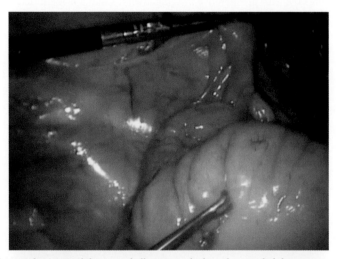

Figure 7-3. Reflecting the terminal ileum medially to start the lateral-to-medial dissection.

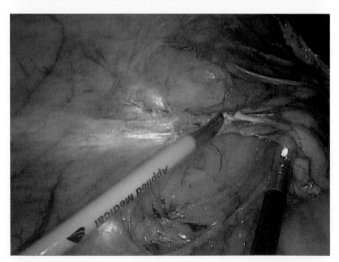

Figure 7-4. Mobilization of the right colon by retracting the cecum medially while dividing the lateral attachment.

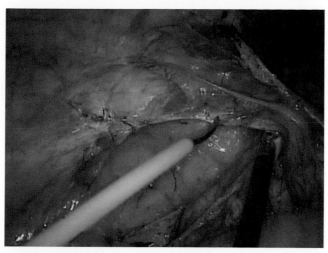

Figure 7-5. Further mobilization of the right colon by retracting the cecum medially while dividing the lateral attachment toward the hepatic flexure.

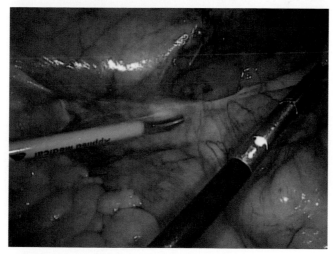

Figure 7-6. Retracting the terminal ileum medially to divide the lateral attachments.

⚠ Pitfalls: The severe inflammatory process in the RLQ, phlegmon, or abscess could distort the anatomy of the ureter by medializing it. To avoid any injury, during mobilization of the terminal ileum, make sure during the mobilization to divide the attachments layer by layer, and when using an energy source, use the jaw of the energy source to dissect the tissues, and then divide what you can see through or when you are certain that there are no other structures involved. Be close to the ileum as you can, to avoid injury to the retroperitoneal structures.

Abdominal Operations

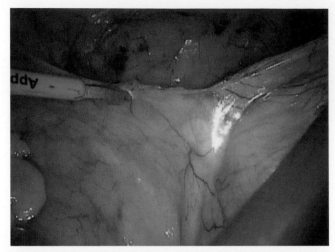

Figure 7-7. Before dividing the lateral attachment of the terminal ileum, assess the anatomy and check the location of the right ureter.

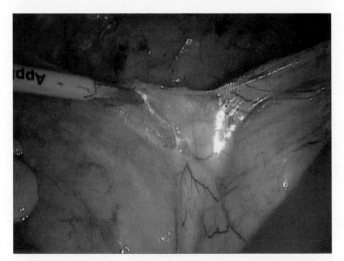

Figure 7-8. Notice that the direction of the dissection is parallel to the right ureter.

- If the inflammation is very severe, and the dissection plane is not clear, or difficult to identify, stop and change the approach. Start from the top down, which allows you to start from a normal anatomical plane and follow it toward the diseased part. The dissection can be started in a normal looking area in the ascending colon or the hepatic flexure (Figure 7-10).

- For hepatic flexure mobilization, place the patient in the reverse Trendelenburg position, and keep the right side up. Use an atraumatic grasper through the suprapubic port, to retract the transverse colon caudally, and the energy source through the LLQ port to dissect. If not possible, especially in high-BMI patients, place an extra 5-mm port in the left upper quadrant (LUQ). In this case, the energy source can by inserted through the LUQ port and the LLQ port can be used for retraction.

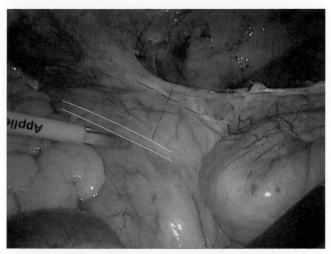

Figure 7-9. Mobilization of the terminal ileum. Notice that the line of dissection (blue dotted lines) are parallel to the right ureter (between two yellow lines) to avoid injury. The dotted red lines represent the wrong direction of dissection, which might lead to ureter injury.

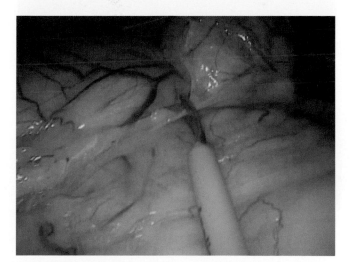

Figure 7-10. Mobilization of the hepatic flexure and the attachments to the gallbladder.

- Using the above configuration, expose the colonic attachments to the liver. Using the energy source, divide these attachments. Again, gentle blunt dissection can be done with the energy source device to drop the colon down, and this will create more space to divide these attachments. This move will help to avoid injury to the colon from the heat from the tip of the energy instrument.

- During mobilization of the hepatic flexure, make sure that you dynamically adjust your left hand that is retracting the transverse colon caudally to provide good retraction (Figures 7-11 and 7-12).

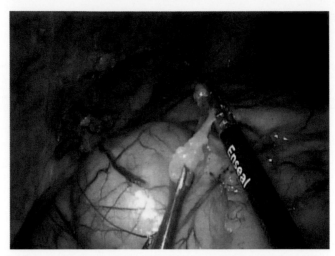

Figure 7-11. Mobilization of the hepatic flexure by retracting the transverse colon caudally, and dividing the hepatic flexure attachment.

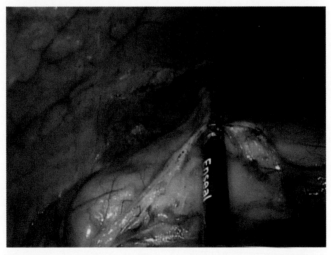

Figure 7-12. Further mobilization of the hepatic flexure by retracting the transverse colon caudally, and dividing the hepatic flexure attachment.

- Apply caution in this step to avoid injury to the duodenum. Avoid manipulating the duodenum, and rather than pushing the duodenum away, take down the filmy attachment and pull the colon away from the duodenum. Be mindful if you need to push the duodenum away that the energy source tip could be hot and this could cause thermal injury.

- After the flexure is taken down, continue with the dissection toward the diseased segment to complete the mobilization of the cecum and the terminal ileum.

- To assess if you are ready for extraction, flip the colon medially toward the midline. It should reflect easily and the Gerota's fascia, and the C loop of the duodenum should be seen, which indicates that the mobilization is adequate. Assess if the mobility of the terminal ileum and the hepatic flexure as well.

- If the planned operation was only ileocolonic resection, without anastomosis, then complete mobilization of the hepatic flexure may not be needed because the division will be at the level of the cecum.

- Prior to making the incision for extraction, make sure that the colon and the small bowel are back to the normal anatomical position. This is important to avoid any twist in the bowel during the extraction and anastomosis. Also, the colon can get tangled with the small bowel if it is not returned to its anatomical position prior to extraction, making it difficult to extracorporealize.

- Use a locking grasper to hold the appendix, and direct the grasper toward the abdominal wall, in the midline, for extraction.

- Desufflate the abdomen, but keep the Trendelenburg position, remove the Hasson trocar, and extend the incision around the umbilicus. Usually extending the incision around the umbilicus inferiorly will be sufficient. If you are planning to construct a stoma, go around the umbilicus toward the left side. This will avoid having the stoma very close to the midline incision. If planning a stoma, then the stoma site can also be used for extraction. An alternate site for extraction is a small Pfannenstiel incision. This has the advantage of minimal risk for incisional hernia development. Intracorporeal division of the mesentery may be necessary to use these sites for extraction.

- Extend the midline incision by dividing the fascia using electrocautery, taking care not to injure any intraperitoneal structure. Place a wound protector, and then use Babcock forceps to hold the appendix or the cecum for extraction. As a general rule, place two Babcocks on the specimen before releasing the laparoscopic grasper. This prevents inadvertent slippage of a Babcock, which can lead to the specimen dropping into the abdomen, especially in morbidly obese patients.

- Exteriorize the cecum and, subsequently, the terminal ileum. If the diseased segment is bulky, it is best to extend the incision. Alternatively, the colon can be divided using a blue load of the GIA stapler, and then tag the distal colon with a 3-0 Vicryl suture that is placed underneath the staple line on the anti-mesenteric side (which will be cut later during the anastomosis) and leave the tails long. Then place a hemostat at the end, and place it back in the abdomen. This will create more space for the terminal ileum to be delivered through the small incision.

- Extra care should be exercised while extracting the terminal ileum, to avoid injury to the mesentery by pulling the specimen. Be gentle, and use your finger to sweep up the terminal ileum and break the suction effect.

- After the specimen is extracted, define the area of proximal resection. In cases of Crohn's disease, define an area that is macroscopically free of any disease, where the small bowel is soft, no creeping fat, and the mesentery is not thickened.

- After the point of proximal resection is defined, run the small bowel to the duodenojejunal junction to make sure there is no other diseased segment. This will identify if there are any obvious strictures. However, small stricture can go unnoticed. A Baker tube can be used and inserted all the way toward the duodenojejunal junction, and the balloon is inflated with saline to 1-cm diameter, and then pulled. This will identify any subtle narrowing in the small bowel (Figure 7-13). It is important to avoid spillage of intestinal contents when doing this maneuver.

- The small bowel from the duodenojejunal junction until the diseased segment that is intended to be resected should be measured and should be documented in the operative report. In addition, if there are any strictures left in situ (with or without strictureplasties), their number and location should be documented.

Abdominal Operations

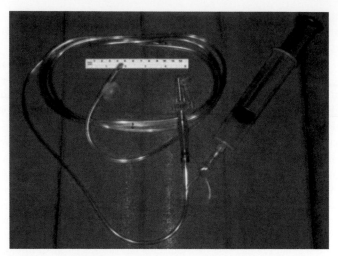

Figure 7-13. Baker's tube, used to identify subtle strictures in the small intestine.

- Divide the mesentery of the small bowel. In this case, the division can be close to the bowel, and high ligation is not required. However, being a little further away from the bowel wall may be easier and reduces chances of postoperative bleeding because the mesentery will not be as thick.

- Score the mesentery using electrocautery superficially. Use Kelly clamps or hemostats to control the mesentery. Please see Chapter 20 for details.

- At this point, the mesentery is divided up to the level of the cecum/ascending colon. The small bowel is ready for division. However, prior to that, distal to the intended site of resection in the small bowel, make an enterotomy and introduce the Baker tube, after it's lubricated in water. Intussuscept the bowel over the tube until the duodenojejunal junction is reached, and then pull it after the balloon is inflated. Pulling the tube should be easy without resistance. If there is, it could be a site for a stricture. Note that the site of the enterotomy that was made for the insertion of the Baker tube is in the "specimen side." As you pull the tube, return the small bowel to the abdominal cavity. This will prevent venous congestion of the bowel because the wound is small, and this will compress on the mesentery. Return the bowel to the anatomical position. After that step is done, divide the small bowel using the blue load of the GIA stapler, including the enterotomy site with the specimen. The specimen at that time can be sent to pathology.

- If the plan is to create an anastomosis, then pull the hemostat that was holding the 3-0 Vicryl suture to deliver the colon back again to the wound. Exteriorize the colon and then align the small bowel and the ascending colon. Make sure there is no twist in the large bowel by following the colon toward the transverse colon. Assess the small bowel, and make sure that the cut edge of the mesentery is straight.

- Prior to making an enterotomy, place a large towel beside the wound, so all the instruments that will be used in the open part of the operation can be discarded after constructing the anastomosis, since it will be contaminated after opening the bowel. All these instruments can be moved out of the operative field after the anastomosis is constructed.

- At that point, make an enterotomy in the antimesenteric side of the small and large bowel using curved mayo scissors. Make sure that it's full thickness and you are inside the actual bowel lumen. Insert the smaller part of the GIA stapler in the small bowel, while placing the other part in the large bowel.

- Align them close together. Advance both parts of the stapler, making sure it is in line with the direction of the bowel so as not to injure the bowel. The assistant should make sure that the mesentery is away, and the staple line will be on the tenia on the colon side. Make sure that the anastomosis is 5 cm or more in length. Fire the stapler, and then open the stapler gently and remove it. Inspect the inside lumen of the bowel to make sure that there is no active arterial bleeding from the staple line. After that, use six Allis clamps to close the lumen of the common enterotomy–colotomy defect, making sure to stagger the staple lines. Use either a blue TA stapler to close the common enterotomy–colotomy. After firing the stapler, divide the tissue beyond the TA staple line, apply Betadine, and release the TA stapler.

- Inspect the staple line for bleeding and make sure that it is intact throughout the whole length of the staple line. Place two stitches at the corner to decrease the tension on the end of the anastomosis between the small bowel and large bowel. After that is done, return the bowel into the abdominal cavity gently. This part may be difficult if the patient's abdominal wall is not completely relaxed. If having difficulty, one should ask the anesthesiologist to make sure that paralysis is complete. Sometimes, it may be necessary to enlarge the incision to safely return the anastomosis back into the abdomen.

- If the omentum can be pulled easily to the wound, cover the anastomosis with omentum, and use a stitch to tie the omentum on the top of the anastomosis as a patch. This stitch can be placed in the mesentery next to the anastomosis or a stitch can be used to bury the corners of the anastomosis and its tails can be used to tie the omentum. Note that tying should be gentle and should not strangulate the omentum.

- All the instruments that were used in the anastomosis should be removed from the operating table because they are now contaminated. Both the surgeon and assistant should change their gloves.

- Reestablish pneumoperitoneum. There are different ways of doing this:
  - First method: loosen the wound protector while the lower end is inside the abdominal cavity, and then place the Hasson trocar without the obturator through the wound protector. Inflate the balloon of the trocar and then twist the wound protector around the Hasson trocar. Use a 0-silk suture and tie it around the Hasson trocar, wrap a wet laparotomy pad around the trocar, and then turn the wound protector again to be snug on the abdominal wall. Prior to turning the wound protector completely, you can place a wet lap around the wound protector and then turn the wound protector over it. This will help prevent air leak.
  - Second method: using a #1 PDS suture in a CT1 needle, close the midline incision in a figure-of-eight fashion. Tie the most inferior sutures, and leave the first and second figure of eight at the upper part of the wound untied. Place the Hasson trocar in between them and then tie them around the Hasson trocar one knot, and then take the two threads and tie each thread around the Hasson trocar in a different direction. Use a hemostat to secure it.
  - Third method: loosen the wound protector, twist it, and apply a Kelly clamp to occlude it completely. It is a very quick way to establish pneumoperitoneum, but the disadvantage is that you will lose the 12-mm access for the Hasson trocar, and you will be left with the 5-mm trocars to finish the operation. A 5-mm camera can be used from one of the lateral ports for final inspection and confirmation of hemostasis.

- Check for bleeding. Make sure that the orientation of the bowel is correct. Suction all the fluids if there is any.

- Remove all trocars under direct supervision.

Abdominal Operations

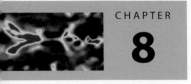

Laparoscopic Sigmoid Colectomy

Preoperative Considerations

Ureteral Stents

In general, ureteral stent placement is not required for routine sigmoidectomy. However, you should consider ureteral stent placement in the following cases:

- Smoldering diverticulitis/phlegmon.
- Presence of active sigmoid inflammation.
- Redo operations.
- Large/recurrent tumor in the sigmoid colon.
- If the computed tomography (CT) scan suggests that the lesion or the pathology is intimately associated with the left ureter.
- Morbidly obese patient.

Imaging

Review the CT scan of the patient very carefully, because it will provide you with a road map to the operation. There are many useful pieces of information that you need to get from the CT scan before you start. These include the following:

- Location of disease.
- Relationship of the diseased segment to the surrounding structures including ureter.
- Nature of splenic flexure including relationship to spleen, pancreas, and surrounding structures.
- Presence or absence of redundancy of sigmoid colon.
- Extent of the disease.

Diverticular Disease

The proximal margin of resection should be a normal colon that should be soft, without muscular hypertrophy and the mesentery should be normal without any thickness. The distal resection margin in these cases will be at the top of the rectum where the tenia converges. In case of diverticulitis, it's important to identify the level of the diseased segment of the colon on preoperative imaging. Diverticulitis usually involves the sigmoid colon. Occasionally, the inflammation is seen in the left colon instead. It is important in this scenario to include the diseased segment and not to limit the resection to the sigmoid colon. Regardless of the proximal extent of resection, the distal resection margin should be the upper rectum.

Occasionally, the upper rectal wall can be very thickened secondary to the diverticulitis, and thus the distal resection could be lower than usual. This will lead to the creation of the colorectal anastomosis lower than anticipated. Typically, this is obvious on a preoperative

CT scan and helps in counseling the patient regarding the possible need for a temporary diverting loop ileostomy. These patients are best served by seeing a stoma nurse and getting preoperative stoma marking for an anticipated loop ileostomy.

Cancer Cases

In all cancer cases, adequate margins are paramount, usually 5 cm of clear margin proximally and distally is sufficient. In addition, the inferior mesenteric artery (IMA) should be divided at its origin to ensure adequate lymph node harvest.

CO_2 Colonoscopy

Intraoperative CO_2 colonoscopy is utilized during sigmoid resections in two stages of the operation.

1. It can be used to identify the distal resection margin when resecting an endoscopically unresectable polyp or a tumor that has not been marked preoperatively with a tattoo and it is not easily identified laparoscopically.
2. It can be used to do the leak test after creation of the anastomosis. Traditionally, a rigid sigmoidoscopy has been used for this; however, the advantage of using a CO_2 colonoscopy are threefold:
   ○ Easy to visualize the anastomosis, and check for:
     ▪ Bleeding.
     ▪ The color of mucosa proximal and distal to the anastomosis.
   ○ If there is bleeding from the staple line, further intervention can be done endoscopically.
   ○ To check the intactness of the circular stapler.

Rectal Washout

We routinely wash the rectum and the sigmoid colon in all cancer cases before we start the case. A 30-French Foley catheter is inserted in the rectum, and then the rectum is washed with diluted iodine. Be mindful to wash the rectum after that with sterile water, especially if you will depend on the flexible sigmoidoscopy to detect a polyp or decide where the distal margin is (Figure 8-1).

Port Sites

Four-Port Diamond-Shaped Configuration (Figure 8-2)

• This configuration will allow you to do any colon or rectal operation.
• A periumbilical port (12 mm) is used for the camera.
• Right lower quadrant (RLQ) port: at the beginning of the case, an atraumatic grasper can be utilized through this port to hold the fat at the level of the sigmoid colon and bring it medially. This port can be enlarged to 10 mm to enable the use of the Endo GIA during resection of the sigmoid colon.
• Suprapubic port: dissecting instruments can be used through this port to mobilize the sigmoid colon and the descending colon. Laparoscopic scissors, hook, or energy source can be used.
• Left lower quadrant (LLQ) port: the initial dissection can be started with the above three ports. However, this port can be used later on during the case during mobilization of the splenic flexure. Dissecting instruments such as a laparoscopic hook, scissors, or energy source can be used through this port to take down the splenic flexure. To retract the colon, an atraumatic

Abdominal Operations

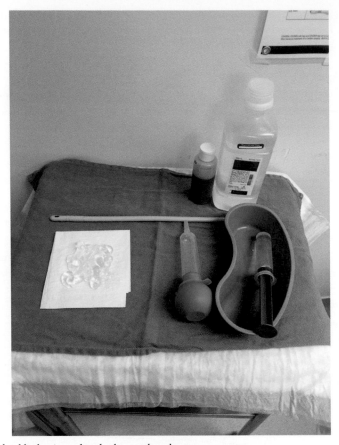

Figure 8-1. Back table that is used to do the rectal washout.

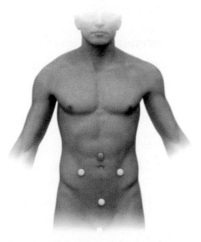

Figure 8-2. Four-port diamond-shaped configuration. The red circle represents a 12-mm site for the camera, and the rest of the ports are 5-mm ports.

grasper can be utilized through either the suprapubic port, or the RLQ port. In obese patients, long instruments may be needed if you are utilizing the suprapubic or RLQ ports to retract to help with splenic flexure mobilization. Also, this port is helpful if there is a second assistant who can hold the mesentery of the sigmoid colon in order for surgeon to do the medial-to-lateral dissection.

Common to All Approaches

- Explore the abdominal cavity for ascites, peritoneal deposits.
- Visualize the liver to check for metastatic lesions in cancer cases.
- Reflect the omentum above the transverse colon.
- Position the OR bed in the Trendelenburg position, and left side up.
- Reflect the small bowel out of the pelvis to the right abdomen.
- Identify the location of the pathology. In cancer cases, make sure you follow the "no-touch technique." In the case of distal sigmoid cancer, mobilization of the sigmoid maybe necessary to visualize the lesion.

Three Approaches to Performing a Laparoscopy Sigmoid Colectomy

1. Medial-to-Lateral

This is our preferred approach, especially in cancer cases.

Advantages

- By starting from the medial approach, the surgeon will benefit from the sigmoid colon attachments that are still in place that are suspending the colon, and this will facilitate the medial dissection.
- Identifying the critical structures (IMA, ureter) at the beginning of the operation.

Limitations

- The medial-to-lateral approach will be technically difficult in obese patients where the mesentery is very thick, making it difficult to identify the IMA.
- If the mesentery is foreshortened in cases of severe inflammation, or diverticulitis, medial dissection is more difficult, and such cases, lateral-to-medial dissection is preferred, especially because ligation of the IMA at its origin is not needed for oncological clearance.
- This technique is not similar to the open technique, and thus, it requires training and practice to recognize the correct planes.

Steps of the Operation

- Identify the important landmarks, including sacral promontory, inferior mesenteric artery, duodenojejunal junction, and the inferior mesenteric vein (IMV).
- Using the RLQ port, hold the mesentery of the sigmoid colon at the midpoint, at the level of the sacral promontory and lift it up toward the abdominal wall. The traction has to be enough to tent the vessel, but not avulse it. A second assistant can hold the mesentery of the rectosigmoid colon while they are standing on the left side of the patient, across the surgeon, while the surgeon can utilize both hands to do the medial-to-lateral dissection.
- Identify the IMA/superior hemorrhoidal.

Abdominal Operations

- Using laparoscopic scissors with an energy source, score the peritoneum along the IMA on its inferior aspect.
- Start the medial-to-lateral dissection by placing the atraumatic grasper underneath the IMA through the RLQ port. Through the suprapubic port, use an atraumatic grasper to drop down the retroperitoneal structures. (Hint: "purple stuff" goes down.)
- Identify the left ureter and left gonadal vessels. After you identify them, bluntly push them down. Continue with the dissection until you reach the white line of Toldt.
- If the ureter is not clear, flip the sigmoid colon medially and start the dissection from lateral-to-medial, just medial to the white line of Toldt. This will facilitate the identification of the ureter from the medial approach. Then resume the dissection from the medial aspect.
- Now focus on the IMA pedicle. Continue the dissection under the IMA until you are close to its origin (3–4 cm cephalad to the bifurcation of the aorta in most patients).
- Clear a window on each side of the IMA close to its origin.
- Make sure that the ureter is identified and dropped down to the retroperitoneum.
- Ligate the IMA proximally and then distally. Then ligate in between, and then divide. Prior to ligation, make sure that the ureter is away. This is a site of ureteral injury.
- Ligation of the IMA can be done by an energy source such as LigaSure, a stapler, or clips.

2. Lateral-to-Medial

Advantages

- This is our preferred approach in all benign cases.
- It's easier to do in cases of severe diverticulitis or any inflammatory process involving the sigmoid mesocolon.
- An easier technique to teach trainees.

Limitations

- After the full lateral-to-medial mobilization of the sigmoid colon and left colon, it will be a bit difficult to divide the IMA because the left colon is now floppy without any attachments. This will be even more difficult if the sigmoid colon is long and redundant.

Steps of the Operation

- Using an atraumatic grasper through the RLQ port, hold the fat at the level of the sigmoid colon at the pelvic brim and pull it medially. Start by using an energy source such as LigaSure or laparoscopic scissors, either with cautery or without, through the suprapubic port to medialize the sigmoid colon. Divide the lateral attachments just medial to the white line of Toldt. Continue with this dissection toward the left colon (Figures 8-3 to 8-9).
- The left hand has a very important role. It should provide adequate traction in the correct direction, to prepare for the mobilization and dissection with the LigaSure using the right hand.
- Take it layer by layer until you reflect the sigmoid colon and its mesentery off the sidewall, the retroperitoneal attachments, and Gerota's fascia.
- Identify the left ureter. It can be found at the base of the sigmoid fossa (Figure 8-10).
- The left hand should apply traction at the same level as the area of dissection.

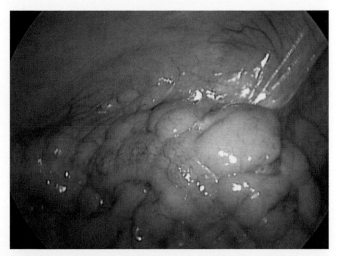

Figure 8-3. Starting the lateral-to-medial dissection at the level of the pelvic brim.

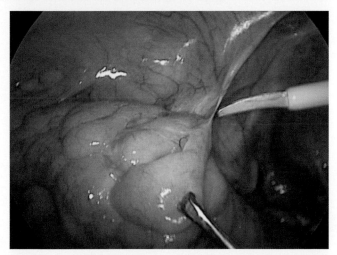

Figure 8-4. Starting the lateral-to-medial dissection by holding the fat and retracting it medially using an atraumatic grasper or, as in the image, a laparoscopic Babcock forceps, and using an energy device with the right hand, and starting the dissection just medial to the white line of Toldt.

⚠ Pitfalls: In a very thin patient, the initial dissection sometimes can be difficult because the planes tend to be fused. Try to identify the actual plane; otherwise, you will end up mobilizing Gerota's fascia (Figures 8-11 to 8-15).

⚠ Pitfalls: In very thin patients, the mesentery of the colon will be very thin. Extra care should be exercised during mobilization of the sigmoid colon to avoid making any defect in the mesentery. Loops of small bowel can be just underneath the mesentery and one might cause thermal injury to the small bowel leading to a missed enterotomy.

Abdominal Operations

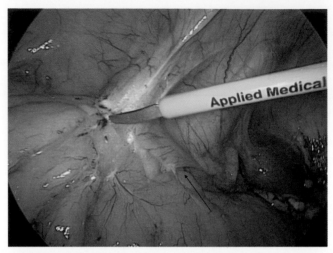

Figure 8-5. Continuing the lateral dissection using the tip of the laparoscopic scissors, which is connected to electrocautery. Notice that the arrow is pointing at the sigmoid fossa, where the ureter can be found.

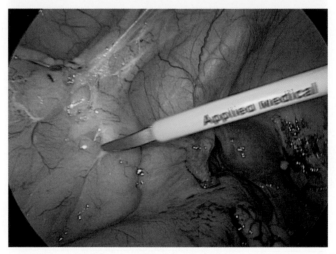

Figure 8-6. Continuing the lateral mobilization. Notice that the white line of Toldt stays with the patient, and the line of dissection is just immediately medial to that line.

- The lateral dissection along the white line of Toldt should be continued until the splenic flexure is reached.
- Grasp the colon at the splenic flexure or the fat close to it, and pull it medially and inferiorly, very gently, and continue with the mobilization.

3. Inferior-to-Superior

This approach is used in cases where the distal margin of resection is defined and there is gross disease of the sigmoid colon making the dissection difficult. The division of the rectosigmoid junction makes it easy to use that as a handle to retract and dissect upward. The surgeon can "hug" the colon and divide the mesocolon thus avoiding injury to the retroperitoneal structures. Classic examples are

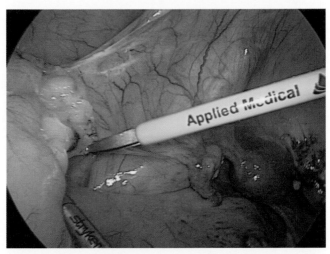

Figure 8-7. Placing the laparoscopic Babcock forceps through the sigmoid fossa and retracting the sigmoid colon medially and using the laparoscopic scissors to continue with the lateral dissection just medial to the white line of Toldt.

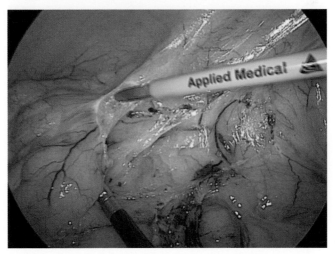

Figure 8-8. Continuing the lateral mobilization. With appropriate traction of the left hand, it will expose the correct plane for dissection.

acute diverticulitis with pericolonic abscess or phlegmon, smoldering diverticulitis with thickened/scarred sigmoid, or cases with diverticular fistulae. This approach can be combined with a lateral-to-medial or a medial-to-lateral approach to complete the sigmoid resection.

Advantages

- This approach is helpful when the normal planes are distorted by severe inflammation (complicated diverticulitis).
- It should decrease the chances (or avoid) injuring any retroperitoneal structures, such as the left ureter, since the dissection is nonanatomical but very close to the colon wall.

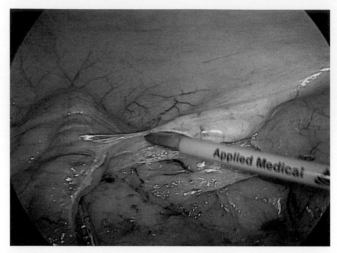

Figure 8-9. Continuing the lateral mobilization along the filmy attachments. The left hand is retracting the colon medially and should be advanced as the dissection progresses to get the best exposure. Notice that after starting the mobilization, the whole instrument is used to retract the colon without grasping anything.

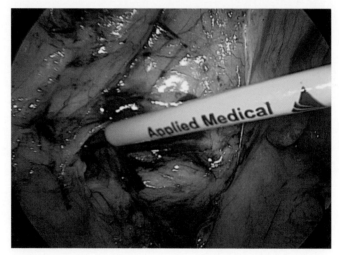

Figure 8-10. Identifying the ureter in the pelvis.

Limitations

- This approach can't be used if the diagnosis is not clear. Meaning that if there is a chance that the pathology could be malignant, then this is not the correct way to do the resection, because this is not an oncological resection, and there will be no enough lymph node harvest since the resection is close to the wall of the colon. In addition, the IMA is not divided at its origin as it is supposed to be done in oncological resection.

Steps of the Operation

- The patient is placed in a maximum steep Trendelenburg position.
- The sigmoid colon and rectum are retracted out of the pelvis.

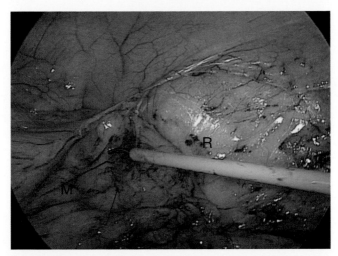

Figure 8-11. Further lateral mobilization of the left colon. Notice here that the dissection was too lateral, and the dissection was lateral to Gerota's fascia (*) that was mobilized. Notice the correct plane of dissection is more medial (arrow). The mesentery of the left colon (M) should be easily separated from Gerota's fascia. R: retroperitoneum.

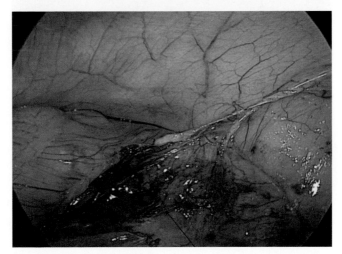

Figure 8-12. Notice that the correct dissection plane (arrow) and Gerota's fascia (*) is dissected from the mesentery of the left colon. It is a common mistake but the most important thing is to recognize it promptly and start the dissection in the correct plane.

- The junction of the rectum and sigmoid is identified by noticing the splaying of the tenia coli. Tactile feedback from the laparoscopic instruments is used to ensure that this area feels normal to determine safe distal margin of resection.

- An energy device is used to create a window underneath the rectosigmoid junction. An Endo GIA stapler with a 60-mm staple is used to transect the rectosigmoid junction. It is critical for the distal margin of resection to be on the rectum and not the sigmoid colon, leaving behind any distal sigmoid colon can lead to a high-pressure anastomosis and will have a higher risk of recurrence in cases of diverticulitis.

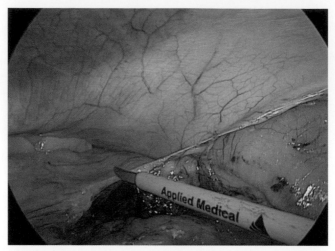

Figure 8-13. Continuing the lateral mobilization of the left colon toward the splenic flexure.

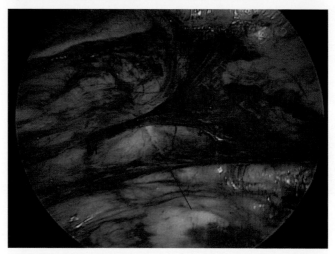

Figure 8-14. This is a clearer dissection plane (arrow) between the mesentery of the left colon (M) and Gerota's fascia (*).

- The distal end of the resected sigmoid can be used as a "handle" to assist in further dissection. This is grasped with a laparoscopic instrument and retracted cephalad. This will expose the mesocolon and the surgeon can continue dividing the mesocolon while remaining close to the colon wall, thus avoiding injury to the ureter and retroperitoneal structures. To perform this step, some medial-to-lateral or lateral-to-medial mobilization may be necessary. Transection of the rectosigmoid junction also helps to find and visualize in the ureters in cases where the sigmoid is grossly inflamed.

Approaches to Splenic Flexure Mobilization

Mobilization of the splenic flexure is necessary in almost all cases to fashion a tension-free anastomosis. There are different approaches to take the splenic flexure down. The surgeon may have to combine different approaches to safely mobilize the splenic flexure mobilization.

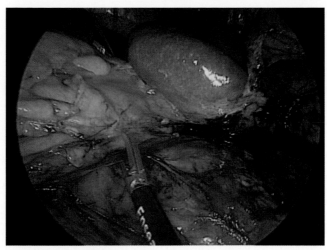

Figure 8-15. Continue the lateral mobilization of the splenic flexure. Be mindful to follow the colon when it turns.

The various approaches are the following:

- Lateral to medial—retrograde
- Lateral to medial—antegrade
- Medial to lateral

Retrograde Approach

- Continue with the lateral-to-medial dissection toward the splenic flexure (Figure 8-13). Once you approach the splenic flexure, it is better to reposition the bed.

- Reposition the bed to the reverse Trendelenburg position. At that time, the operator can stand between the patient legs, and the first assistant stands on the right side. The operator uses an energy source like the LigaSure device through the LLQ port or the suprapubic port, and use an atraumatic grasper either through the suprapubic port or the RLQ port. The assistant can use the RLQ if it is not used by the surgeon and help reflecting the left colon medially. This step may require the assistant to reach their instrument by placing their arm under the surgeon's arm. In patients with a high BMI, or high splenic flexure, long atraumatic graspers sometimes are needed, especially when it's used through the suprapubic port. Alternatively, placing extra ports in the LUQ can help the surgeon to reach the splenic flexure easily.

⚠ Pitfalls: Be proactive in following the colon at the splenic flexure, and make the turn with the colon and continue with the dissection toward the transverse colon. It is easy to continue laterally more than needed. Be mindful that this is a potential area of injury to the pancreatic tail and the splenic hilum. Take these attachments with very gentle sweeps toward the colon and with sharp dissection using electrocautery cautiously, the flexure can be taken down completely. During retracting the splenic flexure to take down the spleno-colic attachment, be very mindful that excessive traction can cause injury to the spleen.

Antegrade Approach

In this approach, the surgeon starts from the transverse colon instead of mobilizing the flexure entirely from below up. It may be particularly useful in patients with a high BMI or a high splenic flexure.

- Position the bed to the reverse Trendelenburg position with the left side up.
- Start from the mid part of the transverse colon and dissect toward the splenic flexure. Identify the transverse colon and hold it with an atraumatic grasper with your right hand through the suprapubic port. The assistant stands to the right of the surgeon and holds the camera.
- The surgeon can use both the suprapubic port and the RLQ port to divide the gastrocolic ligament and enter the lesser sac. The LLQ port can be used as well, by a second assistant, if available, who should stand on the left side of the patient, opposite side of the surgeon, and help with holding the transverse colon and pulling it caudally. Visualization of the posterior stomach wall confirms entry into the lesser sac. The surgeon can then continue dividing the gastrocolic ligament and proceed towards the spleen.
- Once close to the splenic flexure, it helps to tilt the bed to the right and retract the descending colon medially and the transverse colon inferiorly to demonstrate the "knuckle" of the flexure. This can then be mobilized by staying close to it and avoiding injury to the splenic hilum and tail of the pancreas.
- Once this is accomplished, lateral-to-medial mobilization from the splenic flexure down to the descending colon can be carried out. Thereafter, the colon is retracted medially and inferiorly and any embryological attachments to the retroperitoneum and the pancreas are divided. It is important to avoid injury to the mesocolon during this step.

⚠ Pitfalls: Be mindful of the heat spread while doing this step. You can use half a burn or even use only the cut option without using an energy source in the avascular plane to avoid thermal injury.

- If you want to include the omentum with the specimen, identify the stomach and hold it up, and then start dividing just beside the stomach toward the splenic flexure.

⚠ Pitfalls: Be mindful not to injure the posterior wall of stomach while you are doing this. Also, by this approach, you will include all the omentum until you reach the spleen. This could increase the risk of splenic injury.

Medial-to-Lateral Approach

- Using an extra 5-mm port in the RUQ will be helpful.
- Place the bed in the Trendelenburg position, with the left side up. Reflect the small bowel to the right and to the pelvis. This will allow identification of the duodenojejunal junction, transverse colon, and the IMV.
- Reflect the transverse colon cranially, until you identify the IMV, which will be at the inferior border of the pancreas, just lateral to the ligaments of Treitz.
- Apply gentle traction on the vein and then score the peritoneum using an energy source.

- After the peritoneal layer is scored, use an atraumatic grasper to left up the IMV gently, while with the other hand, start with the medial dissection by pushing the retroperitoneum down.
- The dissection is continued caudally toward the IMA, and laterally toward the white line of Toldt, and cranially toward the inferior border of the pancreas (Figures 8-16 to 8-19).

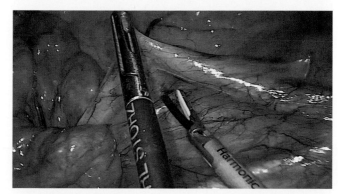

Figure 8-16. Holding the IMV upward, while scoring the peritoneum underneath it with an energy device.

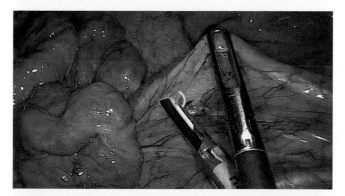

Figure 8-17. Scoring the peritoneum just underneath the IMV from the duodenojejunal junction.

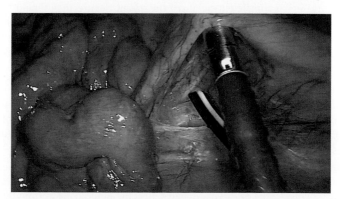

Figure 8-18. Starting the medial dissection bluntly by sweeping the retroperitoneum down and lifting up the IMV, and the mesentery of the colon.

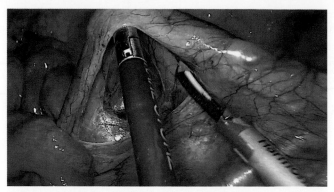

Figure 8-19. The medial dissection should be continued until the white line of Toldt is reached.

> ⚠ Caution: During the medial dissection cranially, a large pulsating vessel will be clear, which is the left renal artery.

- Most of this dissection is done bluntly.
- After that is done, use the LigaSure to coagulate the IMV vein proximally just underneath the inferior border of the pancreas and then distally. Coagulate the vein in between and then divide.
- To enter the lesser sac from the inframesocolic approach, reflect the transverse colon cranially. Lift up the mesentery of the distal transverse colon. Entering the lesser sac should be at a distance 2.5 cm superior to the transverse mesocolon and 2.5 cm lateral (roughly).
- Use an energy device to enter the lesser sac. Once you enter the lesser sac, the back of the stomach is identified. Reflect the stomach up, and continue with the dissection toward the splenic flexure.
- Join the dissection planes together where you have started the medial approach and the lesser sac.

Continue with the dissection until you reach the white line of Toldt. At that stage, you can start from the lateral approach.

- Once the surgeon has completely mobilized the splenic flexure, they should hold the cut edge of the colon and bring it down to the pelvis in order to find any tethering points. Such tethering points, once identified, can be divided. One has to be cautious if such a point is at the mesocolon. Division of the mesocolon has to be done close to the retroperitoneum away from the colon in order to avoid damaging the marginal artery.
- Consider the following points, if the indication for resection was diverticulitis.
  - In case of severe diverticulitis where the plane is not clear, one can use the inferior to superior approach or start from a normal plane by going proximal to the area of pathology and start the dissection from that point toward the splenic flexure. Mobilize the left colon and the splenic flexure, and then go back to the area of pathology.
  - When there is severe inflammation or phlegmon, use a combined technique including electrocautery and blunt dissection using the suction–irrigation device or laparoscopic peanuts "Kittner" to dissect the diseased area and reflect the sigmoid colon from the left side pelvic wall. The dissection in these cases is mainly blunt, with minimal use of electrocautery. The reason is that with the blunt dissection, if it was done in the "correct" plane, it will open up.

But it wound not open up if it was in the wrong plane. If the electrocautery is used a lot in this situation where there is a lot of inflammation and the normal plain is distorted, it will open "wrong" planes easily. Be cautious.

Division of the Sigmoid Colon

- Identify the distal resection margin. In case of diverticulitis, this should be at the top of the rectum. In cancer cases, make sure that the distal resection is below the tumor and there is enough free distal resection margin.

- Score the mesentery at the level of the resection on both sides with laparoscopic hook, or using the tip of the laparoscopic scissors connected to electrocautery.

- Start by dividing the mesentery at the level of the distal resection margin using an energy device such as the LigaSure until the rectum is completely dissected out in preparation for stapling. Alternatively, you can start from the bare area in the mesentery of the sigmoid or at the level of the proximal margin and start dividing the mesentery very close to the sigmoid colon. Continue with dividing the mesentery until you reach the top of the rectum. This is considered a nononcological resection since we are "hugging" the colon and dividing the mesentery just close to the wall, and this technique shouldn't be used in cancer cases, or if there is a suspicion of cancer.

Stapling

There are two options:

- Use the supraumbilical port for stapling. Exchange the 10-mm camera with a 5-mm camera, and place it in the RLQ port. Place the Endo GIA stapler through the supraumbilical port to divide the top of the rectum. The assistant should help using the RLQ and suprapubic ports to help bring the colon through the stapler. This method can be used because the stapling will be at the level of the rectosigmoid junction. However, if the resection will be lower than that, then this is not the optimal way of stapling because the visualization will be more difficult.
  - Advantage: No need to upsize any ports.
  - Disadvantages: Technically more difficult, the quality of the 5-mm camera is not as good as the quality of the 12-mm camera, and the position of the camera from the RLQ will not provide an excellent view as if it was in the supraumbilical port.
- Stapling through the RLQ port: Remove the 5-mm trocar in the RLQ, and extend the incision. Place a 12-mm trocar in the RLQ where the previous whole in the fascia is. Keep the camera at the supraumbilical port. The angle for stapling from this approach is easier; however, the trocar site needs to be closed at the end of the case.
  - Advantages: Better visualization since the camera will be in the supraumbilical port. Ergonomically better, since the surgeon can use the suprapubic port to manipulate the bowel and use the stapler through the RLQ port.
  - Disadvantages: The fascia of the upsized RLQ port site needs to be closed. It is difficult to close it in high-BMI patients, especially when the skin incision is small. A suture passer can be used to close the fascial defect laparoscopically. Alternatively, extend the skin incision more, and use the index finger to feel where the fascia is, and then use a Kocher clamp to grab the fascia to facilitate the closure. A J needle can be used to close the fascia in thigh tight space.

Typically, a medium/thick reload (3.5 mm) is used to divide the sigmoid colon.

- If the mesentery is not divided yet, then from the level where the bowel is divided, start using an energy source and divide the mesentery until you reach the proximal resection margin.

Abdominal Operations

- Place a locking grasper (such as Davis and Geck) on the staple line to prepare for extraction.

⚠ Caution: Prior to extraction, make sure that the small bowel is not lateral to the colon; otherwise, it will prevent adequate extraction of the colon. Also make sure that the colon is completely mobilized in order for adequate exteriorization.

- Extend the periumbilical incision; 2.5 to 3 cm is usually sufficient. You can go around the umbilicus either right or left depending on if you are planning to create an ileostomy or colostomy. Make sure to make the incision on the opposite to the side of the planned stoma. Place your index finger on the top of the umbilicus, and divide the skin just around the index finger to keep the incision as close to the umbilicus as possible.
- Place a medium-sized wound protector. Make sure to sweep with your index finger underneath the ring inside the abdomen to make sure there is no small bowel or other structures are caught between the abdominal wall and the wound protector. Do this step before you pull on the wound protector and turn it.
- Underneath the medium-sized wound protector, place a few laparotomy pads to protect the skin to avoid any contamination to the wound.
- While you are guiding the Davis and Geck graspers toward the abdominal wall, use a Babcock forceps to grasp the staple line and exteriorize the colon. This maneuver must be done by the same individual to maximize the tactile feedback and minimize chances of error.
- Place a small drape or a towel on the lower abdomen beside where you are working. This will be the drape where all the instruments that will be used during creating the purse string will be put on at the end; it should be completely removed from the operative field at the end of this step and should not be reused again at any stage in the operation.
- Identify the proximal resection site. In case of cancer, make sure an adequate proximal margin is achieved, at least 5 cm proximal to the tumor. In the case of diverticular disease, choose an area in the left colon where it is soft, without any hypertrophy of the wall of the colon, and without diverticulosis. If the colon has pandiverticulosis, then make sure the bowel is soft, without hypertrophy, and the mesentery looks normal.
- Apply a Kocher clamp distal to the proposed line of division, and just proximal to it, apply an atraumatic bowel clamp and then divide in between sharply with Metzenbaum scissors, knife, or with electrocautery.
- Send the specimen to pathology.
- Assess the proximal colon vascularity. This is a very critical step because if there is any ischemia, this will contribute to an anastomotic leak.
- Methods to assess colon vascularity:
  - Check if there is obvious pulsatile arteriole supplying the wall of the colon. Occasionally, this is obvious, especially in young thin people.
  - While you are dividing the colon, check the proximal mucosal edges if there is any bleeding. Check the color of the mucosa as well.
  - While dividing the mesentery of the colon. This step is done mostly with LigaSure or any other energy device. However, when you come close to the bowel wall, control the mesentery with hemostats and then divide in between. Release the proximal hemostat temporarily to check for back bleeding. If there is back bleeding, this would be a reassuring sign that this area is vascularized up to that level.
  - Using indocyanine green (ICG) fluorescence imaging.

- Create the purse string suture in the proximal colon in preparation for stapling. This can be done either hand sewn or mechanical.
  - ○ Hand sewn: Start from outside in and continue over and over until you reach the end, and then the last suture should be inside out. Make sure to take full thickness bites, with a little bit of mucosa. Start by taking a bite from inside out, and then continue by taking these bites from outside in, at equidistant points of around 3 to 4 mm, until you reach close to the end, and then when you come closer to the starting point, take the last bite from inside out.
  - ○ Mechanical: Use a reusable auto–purse string suture clamp, where a Keith needle is used to create the purse sting. In this method, one can place the auto–purse string clamp instead of the atraumatic bowel clamp prior to division of the colon.

⚠ Caution: Take small bites of mucosa, otherwise it will crumble.

- Choose the size of the circular stapler, and then take the anvil and dip it in Betadine.
- Place the anvil inside the lumen of the bowel. If the bowel is not wide enough, then use a sponge stick without the sponge to open the lumen of the bowel gently.
- Tie the purse string suture around it securely.
- When you push the knot, make sure to move your hands in a horizontal plane rather than vertical plane to avoid injuring the bowel with the suture itself.
- After you tie, place four knots, and then use the suture to go around the anvil one more time on the opposite side, and your assistant should tie another 4 to 6 knots, and then cut the suture.
- Clear the fat and the extra tissue of the bowel that is in the anvil, to make sure there is no extra tissue between the anvil and the EEA stapler.

⚠ Caution: If there were any diverticula in the bowel at the level of the anvil, then one should cut it out with scissors and use the Baseball-stitch method to place the purse string. If the diverticulum is seen after the fat is cleaned then it can be imbricated with a 3-0 absorbable suture to prevent an area of weakness at the anastomosis.

⚠ Caution: Make sure that the purse string is snug and there is no space between the anvil and the bowel. Gently, you can use the tip of a forceps (like Debakey) to check if there is any space between the anvil and the bowel, which should be tied around snuggly. If there is a space, do another purse string suture and tie it around again.

- Return the bowel to the abdominal cavity.
- At that time, it is advisable that the surgeon and the assistant change gloves, and all the instruments that are used to create the purse string that are kept on the drape should be removed completely from the operative field.
- Establish pneumoperitoneum. There are different ways to do this:
  - ○ First method: Loosen the wound protector while the lower end is inside the abdominal cavity, and then place the Hasson trocar without the obturator through it. Inflate the balloon of the trocar, in case the balloon tipped Hasson trocar is used. Then twist the wound protector around the Hasson trocar. After twisting the wound protector, hold the trocar with your

index and thumb to prevent to unravel the twist of the wound protector around the Hasson trocar. While the surgeon is holding the trocar, the assistant uses a 0-silk suture and ties it around the Hasson trocar. This will establish a seal around the Hasson trocar. Wrap a wet laparotomy pad around the trocar and then turn the wound protector again to be snug on the abdominal wall. This will help prevent an air leak (Figures 8-20 to 8-23).

○ Second method: Close the midline incision using a #1 PDS suture, in a figure of eight fashion. Tie the most inferior sutures, and leave the upper two sutures untied. Place the Hasson trocar in between them and then tie the sutures around the Hasson trocar one knot, and then take the two threads and tie each thread around the Hasson trocar in a different direction. Use hemostat to secure it.

○ Third method: Loosen the wound protector, twist it, and apply a Kelly clamp to occlude it completely. It is a very quick way to establish pneumoperitoneum, but the disadvantage is that you will not be able to place the camera in the supraumbilical area. Place the 5-mm camera in one of the 5-mm ports (such as the RLQ port). This method can be used if the anastomosis is already done, and establishing the pneumoperitoneum is needed only to check for hemostasis or to check for bleeding after removal of port sites.

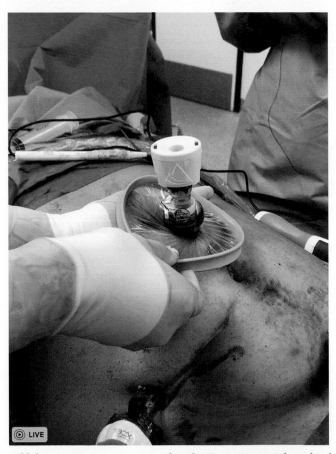

Figure 8-20. To establish pneumoperitoneum again, place the Hasson trocar without the obturator, and place it in the middle of the wound protector, and start twisting the wound protector around the trocar to establish a seal around the trocar.

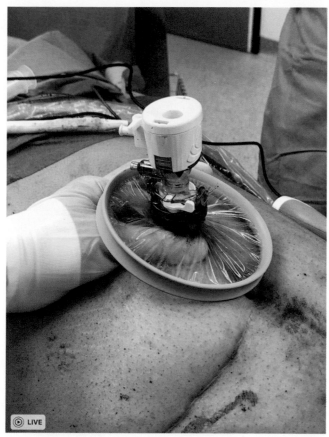

Figure 8-21. After twisting the wound protector around the Hasson trocar to establish pneumoperitoneum, with the left hand, hold it from the middle so the twisting doesn't unravel.

- After establishing pneumoperitoneum, position the bed again to the Trendelenburg position. Assess the abdominal cavity. Identify the anvil.
- Use a laparoscopic Babcock forceps to hold the anvil using the nonmetal portion and pull it gently toward the pelvis. Grasping the metallic part of the anvil with a crushing instrument (like a Davis and Geck grasper) can distort it and lead to failure of coupling of the anvil and the spike.
- Make sure that the reach is adequate and there is no tension at all. If there is any doubt, mobilize more. Mostly, at that time, if further mobilization is needed, further division of the mesentery can be carried out. Make sure when you do this is to stay low in the mesentery to avoid compromising the blood supply of the bowel.
- The first assistant at that time should position themselves between the legs. Carry out a digital rectal examination, followed by placing different sizers. The sizer should be inserted into the anal canal after adequate lubrication. Use the small and medium size and gently negotiate the folds until you reach the staple line. Use the largest size to dilate the anus. Then place the EEA circular stapler. Usually it's either 28 mm or 31 mm.

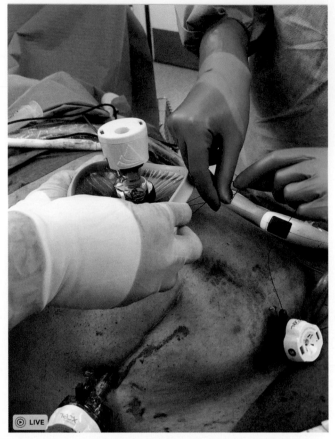

Figure 8-22. While the surgeon holds the Hasson trocar and twists the wound protector to prevent unraveling, the assistant can tie using a silk suture using a sliding knot. After that is tied, place a wet laparotomy pad around the Hasson trocar. Make sure to start by using a Debakey and placing the edge of the laparotomy pad inside the wound, and then turn the rest around the Hasson trocar.

- Make sure that when the stapler is inserted that it effaces the top of the rectal stump (Figure 8-24). If the stump is not fully effaced by the stapler and there is excess tissue in between, it could lead to stapler misfire. Optimally, aim to introduce the spike just above the staple line. It can be introduced just below the staple line as well, but the concern is that the spike can injure the mesorectum and cause bleeding (Figure 8-25).
- Before coupling the anvil with the stapler, make sure to check for the following:
  - No tension whatsoever. At that point, when you couple the two parts of the stapler, you would know for sure if there were any tension. If the colon is straight and taught, don't fire the stapler, and mobilize more.
  - No small bowel going underneath the left colon, and situated in the left upper quadrant. This will be a risk of internal hernia if this is not detected at the time.
  - No twist in the colon. Make sure to follow the cut edge of the mesentery, to confirm that there is no twist.

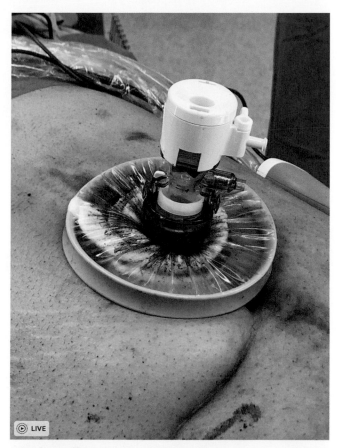

Figure 8-23. Now start the insufflation again.

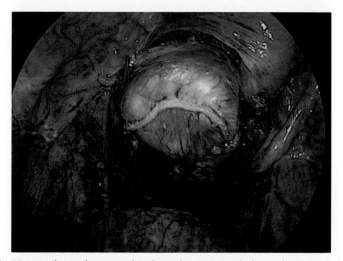

Figure 8-24. The EEA circular stapler is introduced into the rectum and advanced to the end of the rectal stump. Notice that the stapler is fully effacing the rectal stump.

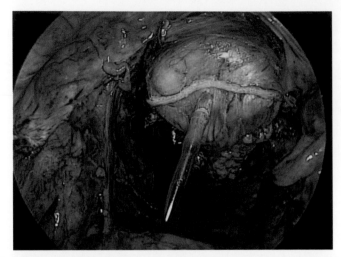

Figure 8-25. The spike of the EEA circular stapler is introduced just posterior to the staple line. Notice the orange color line at base of the spike, this is where the anvil couples with the spike. It is important for this to be clear of any tissues so that the anvil can be coupled without hindrance.

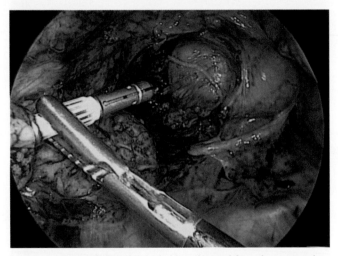

Figure 8-26. Guiding the anvil toward the pelvis by holding the anvil from the nonmetal part.

- Couple the anvil and the spike together. Use an atraumatic grasper, preferably a laparoscopic Babcock forceps and hold it from the nonmetal part and guide it to the pelvis. Gently, you can use an atraumatic grasper, to push the proximal colon as well to assist with coupling (Figures 8-26 and 8-27).
- Make sure there is no tissue apart from the proximal colon and rectum in between the anvil and the circular stapler (Figure 8-28).
- Fire the stapler.
- Follow the manufacturer's instructions for opening of the stapler postfiring.
- With gentle movements that resemble half a circle, withdraw the stapler. Make sure while you are removing the stapler that it is not stuck while you are pulling. Otherwise, it might disrupt the staple line.

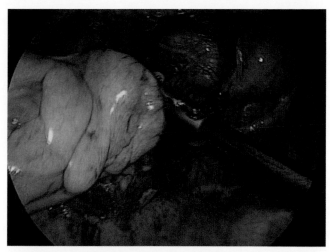

Figure 8-27. Coupling the anvil with the stapler.

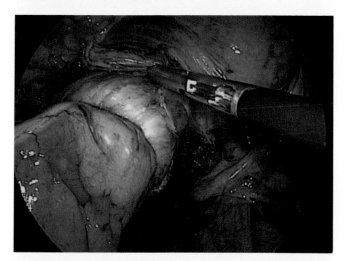

Figure 8-28. During closing with the EEA circular stapler, make sure that no extra tissue that gets in between the anvil and the stapler.

- Leak test: See Figures 8-29 and 8-30.
  - ○ The assistant carrying out the flexible sigmoidoscopy should check the function of the scope and make sure it's adequately functioning (suction, irrigation, etc.) before inserting the scope in the rectum and start insufflating.
  - ○ The pelvis is filled with warm saline. Reduce the Trendelenburg position slightly, to allow the fluids to stay in the pelvis. Use an atraumatic bowel clamp and place it proximal to the anastomosis, to occlude the lumen proximally. It is very important not to pull up on the proximal colon but to push in toward the anastomosis during this step. This will not put tension on the anastomosis and, prevent the air going to the rest of the colon.
  - ○ A CO_2 flexible sigmoidoscope is inserted in the anal canal and advanced to the level of the anastomosis. Endoscopically, check for bleeding from the staple line, the completeness of the staple line, and the color of the mucosa proximal and distal to the anastomosis.

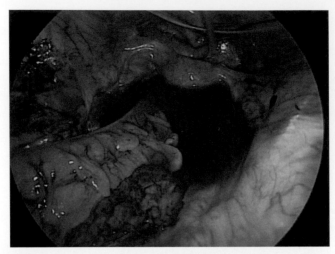

Figure 8-29. Filling the pelvis with saline to prepare for the anastomotic leak test.

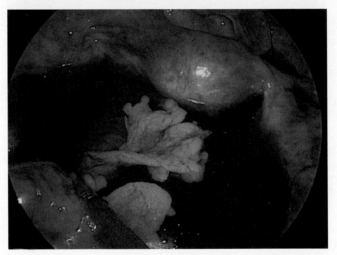

Figure 8-30. Placing an atraumatic grasper proximal to the anastomosis to prevent CO_2 escaping to the rest of the colon and to put tension on the anastomosis.

- ○ If an arterial bleeder is noted, therapeutic intervention such as placement of an endoscopic clip can be done.
- ○ The surgeon at that point should focus on the laparoscopy screen and check for bubbles, and look at the degree of the bowel distension to avoid over distending the bowel, because the assistant at that point is looking at the endoscopy screen.
- ○ Clear communication between the operator and assistance is paramount and can't be over-emphasized during stapling and testing for leak.
- ○ Alternatively, a rigid sigmoidoscopy can be used to insufflate and do the leak test. The advantage of this technique is that it's quick, and a rigid sigmoidoscope is usually readily

available in the OR; however, it has few disadvantages. First, the visualization is not as good using a flexible sigmoidoscopy. Second, it is not possible to do any intervention if there is any bleeding from the staple line.

- If there is no leak, then suction all the fluids in the pelvis, and the endoscopist should suction all the gas in the colon.

- If there is a positive air leak:
  - The best course of action is to redo the anastomosis. Especially if the air-leak is significant or the site of leak is not easily accessible.

  - However, if the leak is a small anterior one that can be easily seen and repaired, place a simple suture to close the defect, and redo the leak test to ensure that it is negative. Consider diverting the patient in that situation. Also, consider leaving a drain in the pelvis in this situation.

Abdominal Operations

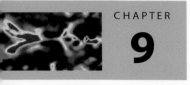

Laparoscopic Low Anterior Resection

Preoperative Considerations

Ureteral Stents

In general, ureteral stent placement is not required in low anterior resection (LAR). However, ureteral stent placement should be considered in the following cases:

- Redo operations.
- Locally advanced/bulky rectal cancer.
- Recurrent rectal cancer.
- If the preoperative imaging suggests that the pathology is intimately associated with the ureter.
- Morbidly obese patient.

Imaging

Review the computed tomography (CT) scan and the pelvic magnetic resonance imaging (MRI) of the patient very carefully, because it will provide you with a road map to the operation. There are many useful pieces of information that you need to get from the CT scan and the MRI before you start.

The following information should be gleaned routinely from preoperative evaluation of the CT scan:

- Location of disease.
- Relationship of disease to surrounding structures including ureter.
- Nature of splenic flexure including relationship to spleen, pancreas, and surrounding structures.
- Presence or absence of redundancy of sigmoid colon.
- Anticipated location of colorectal anastomosis.

An MRI of the pelvis is important to review. The following information should be gleaned routinely from preoperative evaluation of the MRI:

- Location of tumor.
- T stage of tumor.
- Lymph nodal enlargement.
- Distance of tumor from anorectal ring/sphincter complex.
- Involvement of surrounding organs (prostate, seminal vesicles, bladder, ureter, uterus, vagina) or anal sphincters.

- Relationship of tumor to the line joining the sacral promontory to symphysis. pubis. Any tumor below this line is in the true pelvis. Such tumors should be considered for preoperative chemoradiation treatment if they are T3 or higher or have node-positive disease.

Margins

In all cancer cases, adequate margins are paramount. For upper rectal cancer, getting adequate margins is not difficult and we aim for a 3–5 cm distal margin. In mid-to-low rectal cancers, 1–2 cm of negative distal margin should be ideal but 0.5–1-cm margins are acceptable. However, for sphincter preservation, we perform an intraoperative frozen section and aim for microscopically negative margins. If the tumor is very low, and a negative margin cannot be achieved, abdominoperineal resection should be done. In addition, during the resection of the mesentery, the inferior mesenteric artery (IMA) should be divided at its origin. This maximizes colonic reach for a low anastomosis and ensures adequate lymph node harvest.

Prior to starting the case, carrying out the digital rectal examination is important. Not uncommonly, you will find the lesion lower that you initially thought. Do a vaginal exam as well to make sure there is no involvement to the posterior wall of the vagina.

CO_2 Colonoscopy

An intraoperative CO_2 colonoscopy is utilized during LAR in two stages of the operation.

1. It can be used to identify the distal resection margin when resecting an endoscopically unresectable polyp or a tumor that has not been marked preoperatively with a tattoo.
2. It can be used to do the leak test after creation of the anastomosis. Traditionally rigid sigmoidoscopy has been used for this; however, the advantage of using a CO_2 colonoscopy is twofold:
   - Easy to visualize the anastomosis, and check for bleeding and the color of mucosa proximal and distal to the anastomosis.
   - If there is bleeding, further interventions (such as clip placement) can be done endoscopically.
     Occasionally, when the anastomosis is low and there is an air leak identified on colonoscopy, one can place laparoscopic stitches while maintaining colonoscopic visualization to guide the placement of stitches. Of course, in situations where adequate length is available, it is best to revise the anastomosis when air leak is detected.

Rectal Washout

We routinely perform rectal washout in all left-sided and rectal cancer cases. A size 30-French red rubber catheter, or alternatively, a Foley catheter, is inserted in the rectum, and then diluted iodine is instilled in the rectum. While instilling the iodine, the catheter should be elevated above the level of the bed, and then lowered down to evacuate the rectum. We use sterile water to dilute the betadine because it is tumoricidal (Figure 9-1).

Position of the Patient

The patient should be placed in the lithotomy position, as discussed in Section 1 of this book.

Port Sites

Four-Port Diamond-Shaped Configuration (Figure 9-2)

- This configuration will allow you to do any colon or rectal operation.

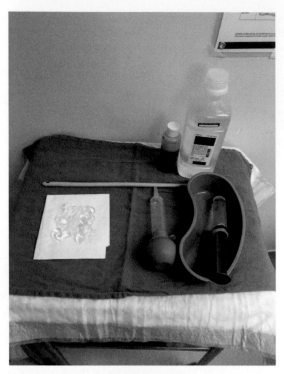

Figure 9-1. Back table equipped to do the rectal washout.

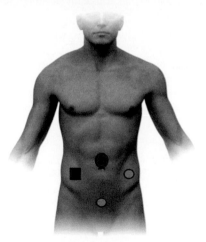

Figure 9-2. Diamond-shaped configuration for the port placement. The RLQ port is a 12 mm port for stapling, 12-mm supraumbilical Hasson port for the camera, and the others are 5-mm ports.

- A periumbilical port (12 mm) is used for the camera. This incision can be extended proximally and distally to extract the specimen.
- Right lower quadrant (RLQ) port: At the beginning of the case, an atraumatic grasper can be utilized through this port to hold the fat at the level of the sigmoid colon and bring it medially in the case of a lateral-to-medial approach. This port can be enlarged to 10 mm to enable the

use of the Endo GIA during resection of the rectum. In the medial-to-lateral approach, this port can be used by placing an atraumatic grasper to hold the mesentery of the sigmoid colon at the level of the promontory and expose the IMA.

- Suprapubic Port: Dissecting instruments can be used through this port to mobilize the sigmoid colon and the descending colon. Laparoscopic scissors, hook, or an energy source can be used. Later during the case, the energy source can be used from this port to do the rectal dissection.

- Left lower quadrant (LLQ) port: The initial dissection can be started with the above three ports. However, this port can be used later on during the case during mobilization of the splenic flexure, especially if the patient's body mass index (BMI) is high, or the splenic flexure is high, then using taking the flexure down through the above three ports will be difficult. Adding the LLQ port will help.

- A dissecting instrument such as a laparoscopic hook, scissors, or an energy source can be used through the LLQ port to take down the splenic flexure. To retract the colon, an atraumatic grasper can be utilized through either the suprapubic port, or the RLQ port. In high-BMI patients, another thing to consider is to use long instruments that are used in bariatric procedures.

- In addition, this port can be an assistant port during the rectal mobilization by retracting the rectum out of the pelvis or lifting up the anterior peritoneal reflection. In addition, it can be used to lift the mesentery of the sigmoid colon upward, and help the surgeon carry out the medial dissection and IMA takedown.

Key Steps of the Operation

This operation can be divided into major steps that need to be accomplished. It is important to view the operation in steps and monitor how much time is spent in each step of the operation.

1. Establish pneumoperitoneum, insert all ports under direct vision, explore the abdominal cavity, provide adequate exposure by retracting the small bowel and sigmoid out of the pelvis, and identify the site of the tumor.
2. Mobilize the left colon and sigmoid colon.
3. Divide the IMA and inferior mesenteric vein (IMV).
4. Splenic flexure mobilization.
5. Rectal dissection (total mesorectal excision) and division.
6. Colorectal/coloanal anastomosis and leak test.
7. Possible diverting loop ileostomy.

Steps of the Operation

Common to All Approaches

- Explore the abdominal cavity for ascites and peritoneal deposits.
- Visualize the liver to check for metastatic lesions in cancer cases.
- Reflect the omentum above the transverse colon.
- Position the operating room (OR) bed to the Trendelenburg position, left side up. Reflect the small bowel out of the pelvis to the right abdomen. Try not to grasp the small bowel, if possible, and use the whole instrument shaft and place it underneath the whole mesentery of the small bowel then reflect it out of the pelvis toward the right upper quadrant (RUQ), until

Abdominal Operations

you expose the duodenojejunal junction. The adequate exposure should allow you to see the pelvis, sacral promontory, IMA, and duodenojejunal junction

- Identify the location of the pathology. In cancer cases, make sure you follow the "no-touch technique."

- Identify the anatomic landmark, including the sacral promontory, right ureter, and the iliac vessels (it can be identified in thin patients).

- There are two approaches, lateral to medial, or medial to lateral. The surgeon can choose either approach; however, in our practice, lateral to medial is preferred for benign pathology and if the sigmoid mesocolon is thickened or foreshortened. The medial-to-lateral approach is preferred for cancer cases.

Lateral-to-Medial Approach

- Position the OR bed in the Trendelenburg position, and tilt the bed to the right side (left side up).

- Identify the site of the pathology.

- Using an atraumatic grasper through the RLQ port, hold the fat at the level of the sigmoid colon at the pelvic brim and pull it medially (Figure 9-3). Start by using laparoscopic scissors, either with cautery or without through the suprapubic port to medialize the sigmoid colon (Figure 9-4). Divide the lateral attachments just medial to the white line of Toldt. Continue with this dissection toward the left colon.

- Identify the left ureter. It can be found at the base of the sigmoid fossa (Figure 9-5). If a ureteral stent is placed, it can be felt as well, even laparoscopically.

- The dissection should be carried out layer by layer until you reflect the sigmoid colon and left colon and its mesentery off the sidewall, the retroperitoneal attachments, and Gerota's fascia (Figure 9-6).

- During mobilization, the retroperitoneal attachments goes down, which are usually purple in color. Pay attention to the difference in the yellow colon between Gerota's fascia, which is pale yellow, and the mesentery of the bowel, which is dark yellow. The plane of dissection should be in-between (Figure 9-7).

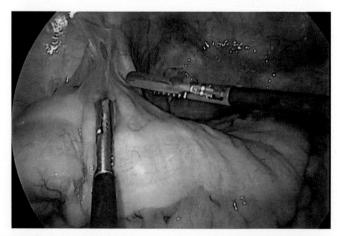

Figure 9-3. Starting the lateral-to-medial dissection by retracting the colon to the midline, and starting to release the lateral attachments.

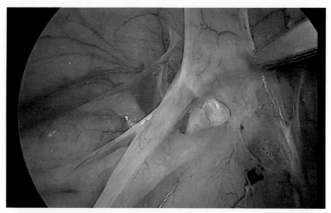

Figure 9-4. Dividing the attachment from the pelvic sidewall. This is the intersigmoid fossa, and the left ureter will be found deeper to this layer.

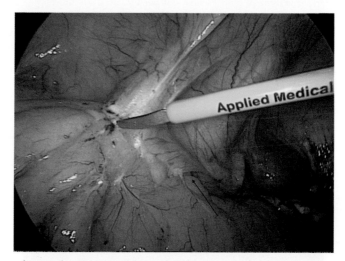

Figure 9-5. Arrow showing the intersigmoid fossa. The left ureter is in the base of the intersigmoid fossa.

- If the plane is not clear, continue with the dissection proximally in a virgin plane, until a good proper plane is established and then return back to the area where the plane is not clear.
- The dissection should be continued proximally until the splenic flexure is reached (Figure 9-8). Continue with the dissection as far as it is possible. When there is no more dissection that can be done from the position (i.e., Trendelenburg position), then go distally again to ensure complete mobilization of the left colon and sigmoid colon.

⚠ Pitfalls: In a very thin patient, the initial dissection can sometimes be difficult because the planes tend to be fused. Try to identify the actual plane; otherwise, you will end up mobilizing Gerota's fascia.

Abdominal Operations

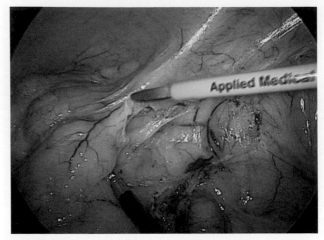

Figure 9-6. Lateral mobilization of the sigmoid colon by retracting the colon medially with the left hand using an atraumatic instrument, and using an energy source to divide the lateral attachments.

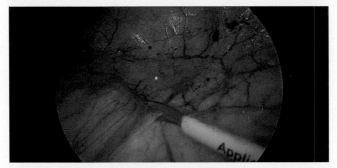

Figure 9-7. Dividing the remaining lateral attachments using laparoscopic scissors between the mesentery of the left colon and Gerota's fascia. Notice the difference in color between the retroperitoneum (*) and the mesentery of the left colon.

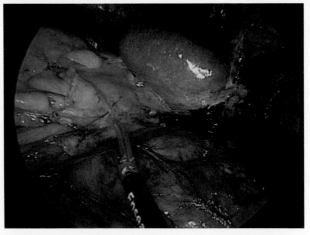

Figure 9-8. The dissection should be continued until the splenic flexure is reached.

⚠ Pitfalls: In very thin patients, the mesentery of the colon will be very thin. Extra care should be exercised during mobilization of the sigmoid colon to avoid making any defect(s) in the mesentery. Loops of small bowel can be just underneath the mesentery and one might cause thermal injury to the small bowel leading to a missed enterotomy.

Medial to Lateral

- Identify the important landmarks, including sacral promontory, IMA, IMV, and the duodeno-jejunal junction (Figure 9-9).

- The second assistant on the patient's left side uses an atraumatic grasper through the LLQ port to hold the mesentery of the sigmoid colon at the midpoint between the bowel and root of mesentery and lifts it up toward the abdominal wall.

- This maneuver will create a "Critical Angle" where the IMA is 60–90° from the horizontal plane of the peritoneum where the division is intended to be (See https://www.sages.org/video/ima-set-up-and-splenic-flexure-release-b-laparoscopic-pg-mis-colorectal-surgery). This angle will be compromised in case of phlegmon or abscess that prevents safe and adequate medial-to-lateral dissection and, consequently, the inability to identify the left ureter.

- Identify the IMA. In obese patients, it might be difficult to visualize.

- In patients with a redundant sigmoid colon, make sure that the redundant sigmoid is pulled out of the pelvis and then work to identify the IMA. Reflect the small bowel away from the pelvis.

- Identify the landmarks prior to starting the medial dissection, including the IMA, the right iliac vessels.

- Score the peritoneum using laparoscopic scissors connected to electrocautery or a laparoscopic hook from the sacral promontory to the duodenojejunal junction.

- The area to be scored should be a few millimeters above the retroperitoneum. Lifting up the sigmoid mesocolon moving it up and down and will help to identify the line where the

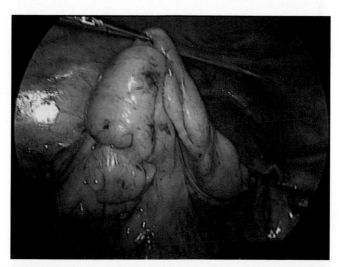

Figure 9-9. Starting the medial dissection by lifting the sigmoid colon at the level of the sacral promontory to expose the IMA.

Abdominal Operations

mesocolon is joining the retroperitoneum, and that line should be the plane of dissection. The mesocolon will move up and down; however, the retroperitoneum will be fixed.

- Score the peritoneum using a laparoscopic hook or scissors. We prefer not to use a sealing device because it will fuse the planes. The wider the window you make, the dissection will be easier, because it will allow better visualization of the left ureter, and gonadal vessels, and avoid creating a tunnel to find these structures.

- Through the suprapubic port, use an atraumatic grasper to start the medial dissection, and separate the plane between the IMA and retroperitoneum. Drop down the retroperitoneal attachments gently following an arc movement from 12 o'clock to 6 o'clock (C or reverse C motion). Usually, all the purple areolar tissue belongs to the retroperitoneum and should be dropped down.

- Use a vessel-sealing energy source, skeletonize the IMA pedicle, and clear the fat around it, in preparation for ligation.

- There is a window of thin mesentery on the other side of the IMA pedicle. Divide that so it will allow you to get around the IMA before ligating it (Figure 9-10).

- Identify the left ureter and left gonadal vessels and drop them down. Continue with the medial dissection until you reach the white line of Toldt.

- Now focus on the IMA pedicle.

- Make sure there is a clear window on each side of the IMA, close to its origin.

- Make sure that the ureter is identified and dropped down to the retroperitoneum.

- If the ureter is not clear, then stop, and start the dissection from lateral to medial. It is critical to not divide the IMA prior to identifying the left ureter clearly. If the ureter is not identified, then converting to hand assist or open surgery should be considered prior to ligation of the IMA. Intraoperative stents placement by the urology team can help as well if that is possible. Using an energy source, ligate the IMA proximally close to the aorta, and then distally. Then, ligate in between, and then divide. Make sure that the energy source you are using can control the IMA. In our practice, we prefer LigaSure. If the IMA is not completely ligated with one firing, then when you divide using the LigaSure, don't cut the whole part that is burned (i.e., don't pull the bottom to cut all the way what is in the LigaSure's jaws. Just do a partial cut). By doing this, there will be a sealed stump. Consequently, advance the LigaSure and ligate the rest of the pedicle and then divide. This avoids the pitfall of using the blade in the LigaSure to cut the IMA partially while it's not sealed completely (Figure 9-11).

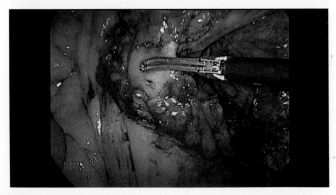

Figure 9-10. After skeletonizing the IMA, division is carried out using an energy source.

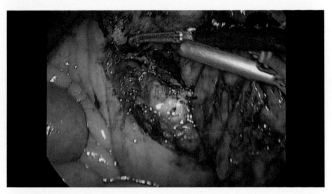

Figure 9-11. The IMA pedicle is divided.

⚠ Pitfalls: Avoid excessive traction during dividing the IMA. Otherwise, avulsion or vascular injury could happen to the IMA. Inform the second assistant to relax while the mesentery of the sigmoid colon is pulled upward, especially during the IMA ligation.

⚠ Pitfalls: In elderly people, the IMA could be atherosclerotic. After dividing the IMA, be ready with an atraumatic grasper to grasp the IMA stump in case there was bleeding due to failure of the energy source or stapler. Prior to dividing the IMA, make sure that an Endoloop Ligature is available in the room, so if you had to grab the IMA stump, you can use the Endoloop Ligature to control the bleeding, since it will be very close to the aorta. The laparoscopic stapler with the vascular load can also be used to secure and divide the IMA if there is enough length to accommodate the breadth of the stapler.

- After that is done, lateral dissection can be started. This dissection will be easy since most of the work is done from the medial dissection.

Approaches to Splenic Flexure Mobilization

Mobilization of the splenic flexure may be necessary to fashion a tension-free anastomosis. There are different approaches to take the splenic flexure down. The surgeon may have to combine different approaches to safely mobilize the splenic flexure. Choosing one approach could depend on the surgeon's experience with that approach, the patient's BMI, and anatomical factors such as high splenic flexure.

The various approaches are:

- Lateral to medial—retrograde
- Lateral to medial—antegrade (supramesocolic approach)
- Medial to lateral

Retrograde Approach

- Continue with the lateral-to-medial dissection toward the splenic flexure. Once you approach the splenic flexure, it is better to reposition the bed.
- Reposition the bed to the reverse Trendelenburg position. At that time, the operator can stand between the patient legs, and the first assistant stands on the right side. The operator uses an energy source like the LigaSure device through the LLQ port or the suprapubic port and uses an atraumatic grasper either through the suprapubic port or the RLQ port. The assistant can

Abdominal Operations

use the RLQ to help reflect the left colon medially. This step may require the assistant to reach their instrument by placing their arm under the surgeon's arm. In high-BMI patients or if the patients are tall, long atraumatic graspers sometimes are needed, especially when it's used through the suprapubic port.

⚠ Pitfalls: Be proactive in following the colon at the splenic flexure, and make the turn and continue with the dissection toward the transverse colon. It is easy to continue laterally more than needed. Be mindful that this is a potential area of injury to the pancreatic tail and the splenic hilum. Take these attachments with very gentle sweeps toward the colon and with sharp dissection using electrocautery cautiously, the flexure can be taken down completely. During retracting the splenic flexure to take down the splenocolic attachment, be very mindful that excessive traction can cause injury to the spleen.

Antegrade Approach (Supramesocolic Approach)

In this approach, the surgeon starts from the transverse colon instead of mobilizing the flexure entirely from below up. It may be particularly useful in patients with a high BMI or a high splenic flexure. The surgeon stands between the patient's legs and assistant stand on the patient's right side. Start from the mid part of the transverse colon and dissect toward the splenic flexure. Identify the transverse colon and hold it with an atraumatic grasper in your left hand through the suprapubic port. The assistant holds the camera and uses the RLQ port to hold up the gastrocolic ligament against the point of the transverse colon being held by the operating surgeon. The operating surgeon divides the gastrocolic ligament via the LLQ post using LigaSure in order to enter the lesser sac. Visualization of the posterior stomach wall confirms entry into the lesser sac. The surgeon can then continue dividing the gastrocolic ligament and proceed toward the spleen. Once close to the splenic flexure, it helps to tilt the bed to the right and retract the descending colon medially and the transverse colon inferiorly to demonstrate the "knuckle" of the flexure. This can then be mobilized by staying close to it and avoiding injury to splenic hilum and tail of pancreas. Once this is accomplished, lateral-to-medial mobilization from splenic flexure down to the descending colon can be carried out. Thereafter, the colon is retracted medially and inferiorly and any embryological attachments to the retroperitoneum and the pancreas are divided. It is important to avoid injury to the mesocolon during this step.

⚠ Pitfalls: Be mindful of the heat spread while doing this step. You can use half a burn or even use only the cut option without using energy in the avascular plane.
   If you want to include the omentum with the specimen, identify the stomach and hold it up, and then start dividing just beside the stomach toward the splenic flexure.

⚠ Pitfalls: Be mindful not to injure the posterior wall of stomach while you are doing this. Also, by this approach, you will include all the omentum until you reach the spleen. This could increase the risk of splenic injury.

Medial-to-Lateral Approach (Inframesocolic Approach)

- Using an extra 5-mm port in the RUQ will be helpful.
- Place the bed in the Trendelenburg position, and tilt the OR table to the right. Reflect the small bowel to the right to identify the duodenojejunal junction, transverse colon, and the IMV.

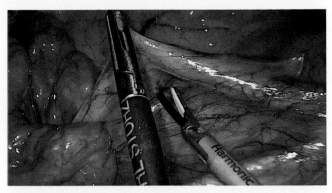

Figure 9-12. Holding the IMV using an atraumatic grasper. Use an energy source to start the dissection beneath the vein.

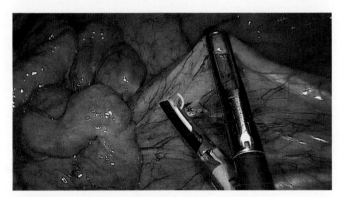

Figure 9-13. Scoring the peritoneum just underneath the IMV.

- After identifying the IMV, apply some traction on the vein and open the peritoneum below the vein using an energy source, in a similar fashion to the medial approach of IMA (Figures 9-12 and 9-13).

- Use the atraumatic grasper to start the medial-to-lateral dissection by dissecting and pushing the retroperitoneal attachments and the attachments of Gerota's fascia down, and separating it from the mesentery of the left colon while advancing the atraumatic grasper until you reach the white line of Toldt (Figures 9-14 and 9-15). The dissection direction should be similar to the IMA dissection, an arc movement from 12 o'clock to 6 o'clock. Some prefer to use gauze to do the dissection to prevent injury to the mesocolon.

- After that is done, there are two techniques to enter to the lesser sac:

  ○ First technique: While still lifting up the IMV, cranially will be the mesentery of the transverse colon. The pancreas can be identified. Dissect the transverse mesocolon from the medial approach just above the pancreas until the lesser sac is entered. Be cautions of the splenic vein while doing this step. Once you enter the lesser sac, the back of the stomach is identified. Continue with the dissection toward the splenic flexure.

  ○ Second technique: Hold the transverse colon just at the level of the IMV. Identify the IMV and choose a point around 2–3 cm above the IMV, 2–3 cm to the left of the duodenojejunal junction, and start dividing. By doing this, a window above the pancreas into the lesser sac is created. Avoid injury to the left branch of the middle colic while doing this step.

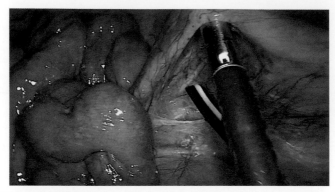

Figure 9-14. Lifting up the IMV, and starting the blunt medial dissection.

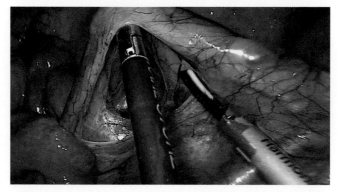

Figure 9-15. Blunt dissection separating the mesentery of the left colon from the retroperitoneum and Gerota's fascia.

- ○ Use the LigaSure to coagulate the IMV vein proximally just underneath the inferior border of the pancreas and then distally. Coagulate the vein in between and then divide in between.
- Join the dissection planes together where you have started the medial approach and the lesser sac.
- Continue with the dissection until you reach the white line of Toldt. At that stage, you can stat from the lateral approach.

Once the surgeon has mobilized the splenic flexure completely, hold the cut edge of the colon and bring it down to the pelvis in order to find any tethering points. Such tethering points, once identified, can be divided. One has to be cautious if such a point is at the mesocolon. Division of the mesocolon has to be done close to the retroperitoneum away from the colon in order to avoid damaging the marginal artery.

Total Mesorectal Excision (TME) Dissection

- The patient should be placed in a steep Trendelenburg position with the right side down.
- In females, if the uterus is large, or bulky, lifting the uterus out of the way will help in the anterior dissection and manipulation of the rectum. Pass a Keith needle through the skin, just beside the suprapubic port, and under laparoscopic guidance, pull the needle, and then redirect to go through the thin part of the body of the uterus, and then push the needle to exit from

the abdomen just beside the point of entrance. Cut the needle and then place a folded 4 × 4 gauze and then tie using a sliding knot on the gauze while you are tying assess if this maneuver is lifting the uterus out of the way (Figures 9-16 to 9-18).

- After the IMA is divided, the assistant who is standing on the left side of the patient should pull the sigmoid colon upward toward the abdominal wall, and out of the pelvis and to the left side using the LLQ port.

- To enter the proper TME plane, start from the divided IMA pedicle and lift up the rectosigmoid upward using the RLQ port by opening the jaws of the atraumatic grasper transversely, and place it posterior to the rectosigmoid. This will help identify the plane of dissection posteriorly. Attempt to identify the hypogastric nerves, and try to push them away prior to starting the dissection.

- Using the suprapubic port, use an energy source, preferably a laparoscopic hook or laparoscopic scissors connected to electrocautery to start the dissection. LigaSure can be used as well; however, it will fuse the planes, and it is easy to be off the appropriate plane without knowing. Using the monopolar cautery is better since it will open the dissection plane, and if the dissection is not in the proper plane, bleeding might be encountered.

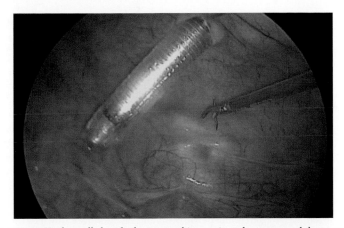

Figure 9-16. Inserting a Keith needle beside the suprapubic port in order to suspend the uterus.

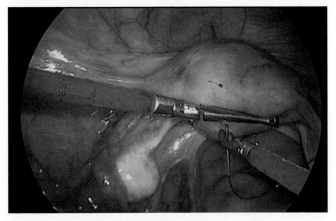

Figure 9-17. Inserting the Keith needle in the body of the uterus.

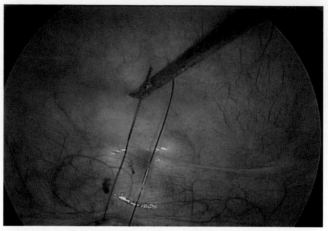

Figure 9-18. Reinserting the Keith needle beside the entry point in the suprapubic area.

- Start the dissection posteriorly with adequate traction and lifting the rectum up and out of the pelvis. The dissection should be in the TME plane, where the foamy filaments (angel hair) are found. The dissection should be continued distally as much as possible (Figure 9-19). The left hand should be adjusted frequently to provide traction and counter traction. The direction of the dissection posteriorly will be like an arc shape. Be aware of the curvature of the sacrum during the posterior dissection, and the direction of the dissection should be adjusted. Otherwise, injury to presacral vessels could happen.

- Then the rectum is pulled to the right side and out of the pelvis, and the operator using the suprapubic port or the RLQ port score the left pararectal sulcus (Figures 9-20 and 9-21). Further dissection is carried out until it's joined with the posterior dissection. Prior to starting this maneuver, check the location of the left ureter. We have already checked the site of the ureter at the level of the pelvic brim, but while you are doing this part of the dissection, make sure that you know the course of the ureter.

- Identify the left ureter again at the pelvic brim and then follow it down to the deep pelvis and make sure while you are doing the lateral dissection, that you are away from it.

- During dissecting the right and left lateral attachments, LigaSure can be used to control the lateral stalks, which contain the middle rectal vessels.

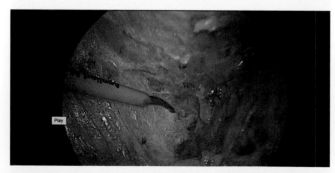

Figure 9-19. In cases when a complete TME is required, the posterior dissection should be continued until the pelvic floor.

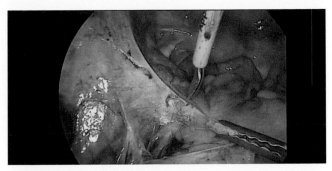

Figure 9-20. Dissecting the left pararectal sulcus by retracting the rectum medially and using the laparoscopic scissors to dissect the plane in between the rectum and left pelvic sidewall.

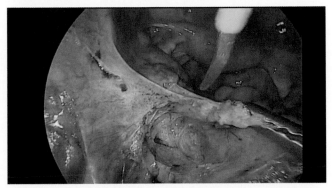

Figure 9-21. Continuing with the dissection in the left pararectal sulcus. Notice that the planes are joined with the posterior dissection plane and the "angel hair" is shown from the left side of the dissection.

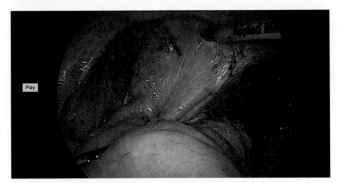

Figure 9-22. Pulling the rectum out of the pelvis and downward to expose the anterior plane, and then scoring the anterior plane at the peritoneal reflection.

- During the dissection laterally and at the time of trying to join this plane with the posterior plane, be mindful not to go too laterally to prevent injury to the structures in the lateral wall of the pelvis.

- The assistant should now pull the rectum out of the pelvis and push it down towards the patient's spine at the same time. The operator using laparoscopic scissors connected to electro-cautery starts with the anterior dissection. Score the peritoneal reflection (pouch of Douglas) anteriorly (Figure 9-22) and then after that, in males, push the seminal vesicles upward and

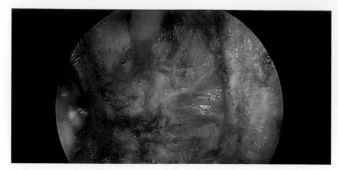

Figure 9-23. In cases of complete TME, posterior dissection should be continued until the pelvic floor muscles are reached.

away from the rectum. Continue with the anterior dissection until you join the planes on both sides with the lateral dissection.

- Determine the level of the resection, in case of a complete TME one has to continue the posterior dissection to the pelvic floor (Figure 9-23). If it was obvious laparoscopically, then continue with the dissection posteriorly, laterally, and anteriorly until you are distal to the lesion. If it is not obvious, flexible or rigid sigmoidoscopy can be used to adequately locate the site of the lesion. If that is done, then the operator can use the LigaSure or laparoscopic scissors to score the mesentery at the level of the lesion to easily identify it during the dissection laparoscopically.

- Once the area is identified, use a LigaSure to clear the mesorectum posteriorly. Using the LigaSure, use the upper jaw of the LigaSure and slide it just posterior to the posterior wall of the rectum and then close the jaws while pulling down and away from the posterior wall of the rectum to avoid causing any thermal injury , and then coagulate the mesentery and divide it. Continue with this maneuver until the rectum is cleared circumferentially in preparation for stapling. A pitfall in this step is to divide the mesorectum distal to the intended area of division. This will lead to devascularization of a part of the rectal stump and could lead to anastomotic leak. So, during division of the mesorectum, all effort should be done to divide the mesorectum in a perpendicular fashion.

Stapling the Rectum (Figures 9-24 and 9-25)

- There are a couple of options to staple the rectum. Usually, an Endo GIA™ stapler purple load (staple height: 3.5 mm) is used. If the level of resection is in the upper rectum, then place the stapler through the supraumbilical port, and replace the camera with another 5 mm, 30 degrees, and insert it through the RLQ port, and then divide the rectum. If the level of resection is low, this maneuver would not be suitable. Then, in this case, keep the camera in the supraumbilical port, and upsize the RLQ port to a 12 mm, and then use it for stapling.

- The stapler should be introduced through the RLQ port. The operator can use the LLQ port to adjust the rectum and manipulate it so the stapler can be applied as close to a right angle as possible. The stapler should be introduced to the right side of the rectum, and then the jaws of the stapler should be articulated toward the left. With the left hand, the rectum should be pulled out of the pelvis and manipulated to facilitate the stapling.

- In cases of a narrow pelvis, stapling the rectum can be very challenging. Consider the following:

  ○ Top-down approach where the stapler is inserted through the RLQ port, but instead of coming from the right side of the rectum, try to staple the rectum from the top of the rectum downward (top-down approach).

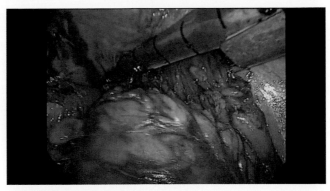

Figure 9-24. Stapling the rectum using an Endo GIA stapler.

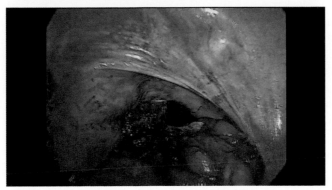

Figure 9-25. Most of the time, two firings of the Endo GIA stapler are required to completely transect the rectum.

- ○ Make sure that the rectum at the level of resection is dissected out and cleared circumferentially.
- ○ During stapling, make sure that the lower jaw is the metal part of the stapler, which will make it easier to slide.
- ○ A second assistant can push the perineum using a fist. This could help as well.
- ○ Instead of using the usual 60-mm length of the purple load (3.5-mm thickness) GIA stapler, consider using the 30-mm length.
- ○ Use the suprapubic port to place the stapler instead of the RLQ port.
- ○ If laparoscopic stapling is deemed impossible, then one can make a Pfannenstiel incision and use a CONTOUR curved cutter stapler to divide the rectum.

Specimen Extraction, Colorectal Anastomosis, and Leak Test

- Place a locking grasper on the staple line of the proximal rectum.
- Prior to extracting the rectum, make sure of the following:
  - ○ That the left colon can reach to the pelvis easily without tension.
  - ○ There is no twist in the colon. You can check that by following the cut edge of the mesentery of the left colon. Also follow the colon itself until the splenic flexure to make sure the orientation is correct.

○ There is no small bowel underneath the mesentery of the colon. Otherwise, it will be difficult to pull the specimen. In addition, if that left in place after the anastomosis without correction, this will lead to internal hernia and small bowel obstruction.

- Extend the periumbilical incision proximally and distally. Place a wound protector; usually the medium size would be optimal. Using Babcock forceps, grasp the staple line, after you direct the locking grasper to the abdominal wall toward the midline incision. Place laparotomy towels just underneath the wound protector. Bring another towel so all the instruments that will be used for the purse string can be put in this towel and removed the operative filed completely and never used again in the operation. Exteriorize the rectum and colon.

- Assess the tumor location, and make sure that there was an adequate distal margin.

- Identify the proximal resection margin. Typically, choose an area in the left colon, just proximal to the IMA pedicle. Make sure there is adequate proximal margin, and the bowel is healthy.

- Divide the mesentery up to the level of the planned resection. Prior to reaching the colonic wall and dividing all the mesentery, use Metzenbaum scissors and divide the remaining mesentery and pericolonic fat to assess for bleeding. If there is bleeding, then most likely the blood supply to the bowel is adequate.

- Place a Kocher clamp distal to the area of planned resection. Place a bowel clamp just proximal to Kocher clamp. Divide in between using curved Mayo scissors

- Send the specimen to pathology. If the distal margin is close, then ask the pathologist to open the specimen and assess the distal margin.

- Create the purse string suture in the proximal colon. This can be done either:
  ○ Automatically by using the purse string clamp, or
  ○ Manually—hand sewn

- To do it manually, use a 2-0 Prolene suture to create the purse string, with hemostat at the end. The first suture should be from inside out, and then, the next bites, from outside in, and continue until the last bite, where you have to go from inside out.

- During suturing, take a little bit of mucosa and lots of submucosal. With the back of the needle, push the mucosa away to minimize the mucosa in the bite, before you take it. Insert the needle perpendicular to the bowel wall. Leave 0.5 cm between each bite. At the end, when you are almost back to the first suture you started with, take the last bite inside out.

- After that is done, use a sponge stick without a sponge to open the bowel lumen. Place the head of the anvil gently inside the lumen. To facilitate the process, the anvil can be dipped in Betadine. The assistant should hold the anvil, while the surgeon should pull the purse string and tie it securely around the anvil. Four knots should be sufficient. Make sure when you tie, that you are tying around a cuff of good tissue that will hold the suture. Then after that, the surgeon would hold the anvil, and the assistant should take the sutures to their side and tie another four knots as well. Make sure there is no gap between the metal part of the anvil and the bowel.

- If there was a gap between the metal part of the anvil and the bowel, do another purse string close to the anvil to make certain that there is no gap between the anvil and the bowel.

- Clear the fat from the colon that is in the "cup" of the anvil to minimize the extra tissues that will be in the stapler during the anastomosis.

- Return the bowel into the abdominal cavity.

- Establish pneumoperitoneum. There are different ways to do that:
  ○ Close the midline incision with a 0-PDS sutures, in a figure of eight fashion, and leave the most proximal sutures untied, and place the Hasson trocar again at the upper part of the wound and use the sutures that are placed in the upper part of the wound to secure the Hasson trocar.

○ Undo the wound protector but keep it in place. Place the Hasson port with the balloon inflated, without the obturator in through the wound protector, and then twist the wound protector around the Hasson while holding the Hasson in the middle of it. The assistant should use a 0-silk suture and tie around the Hasson trocar and the twisted plastic of the wound protector. This will provide an air tight closure between the wound protector and the Hasson trocar. Usually, two sutures are required to make it airtight as one thread tends to break. Then, place a wet lap just underneath the wound protector inside the wound to prevent any air leak and turn the wound protector back again, now, you can re-establish pneumoperitoneum (Figures 9-26 and 9-27).

○ Some wound protectors come with a gel cap. We usually don't use it, but this is another option to establish pneumoperitoneum, to cover the wound protector with the cap designed for it.

• Place the patient again in the Trendelenburg position, and tilt the patient to the right side.

• Prior to stapling, consider doing a leak test to the rectal stump if needed. Most of the time, that step is omitted; however, consider it if there were difficulties with stapling or if you are suspecting that there was an inadvertent injury to the rectal stump during the rectal dissection.

• Identify where the anvil is and direct it toward the pelvis.

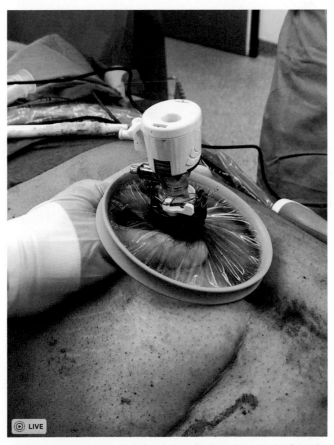

Figure 9-26. Reestablishing pneumoperitoneum by placing the Hasson trocar (without the introducer) inside the wound protector and then holding the trocar as shown.

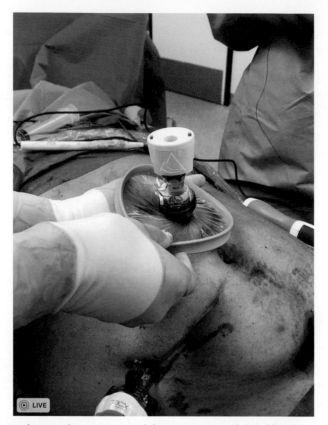

Figure 9-27. Twisting the wound protector around the Hasson trocar while holding the trocar.

- Make sure that there is no tension when you bring the proximal colon with the anvil toward the pelvis (Figure 9-28).
- The second assistant can place lubricated sizers in the rectum. Typically, there are three sizes. Start with the smallest. The sizer would dilate the anal opening and would help the assistant to assess where the stapler will reach in the rectum. Then place the EEA circular stapler.

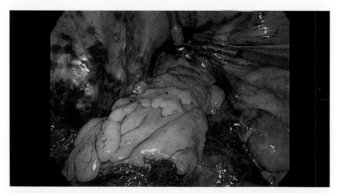

Figure 9-28. Bringing the left colon down to the pelvis to assess for the reach and to checking if there is any tension prior to creating the anastomosis.

Usually, either size 28 mm or 31 mm is used. The stapler size is chosen based on the size of the colon and the compliance of the anus. The stapler should be lubricated, and then inserted in the anal canal. Occasionally, the anus needs more dilatation to accommodate the stapler, especially if size 31 mm is used. Use two fingers to gently dilate the anus, and then insert the stapler.

- Advance the stapler until it reaches the end of the rectal stump, and the stapler "cup" is effaced (Figure 9-29). Make sure that the spike of the stapler will come out in the center of the rectal stump, just above or below the staple line, preferably above it, to avoid causing any bleeding in the mesorectum (Figure 9-30).

- Occasionally, the operator can use an atraumatic grasper and push the rectal stump while the jaws of the instrument open to help the spike to go through the rectal stump. Then the same maneuver can be used until the orange color of the spike can be seen.

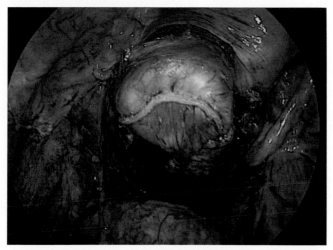

Figure 9-29. Advancing the EEA circular stapler to the end of the rectal stump and making sure that the "cup" of the EEA stapler is fully effaced prior to introducing the spike.

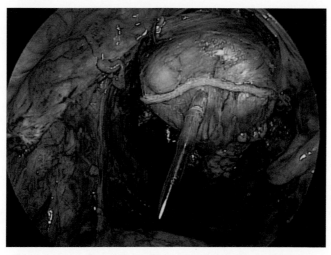

Figure 9-30. Introducing the spike of the EEA stapler just posterior to the staple line.

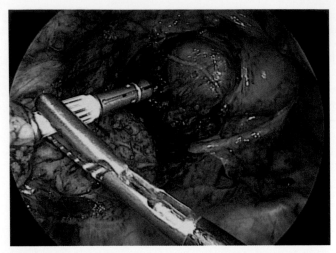

Figure 9-31. Guiding the anvil toward the pelvis to couple with the spike of the EEA circular stapler.

- After that, the surgeon can direct the anvil toward the spike of the stapler and couple the two parts (Figure 9-31).
- Prior to this maneuver, it is critical to make sure of the following:
  - That the left colon can reach down to the pelvis easily without any tension. One way to assess is to hold the anvil and bring it down to the pelvis close to the rectal stump. If there is no tension and the colon is not pulled taught and there is laxity, then it's a good sign there is no tension. Another way, after the colon is brought down to the pelvis, is to leave it and check if the colon retracts back into the abdominal cavity. If it stays in the pelvis, it's a good sign that the colon is mobilized enough; however, if it returned (retracted) back to the abdominal cavity, most probably further mobilization is needed.
  - Make sure there is no twist in the colon. You can check that by following the cut edge of the mesentery of the left colon. Also, follow the colon itself until the splenic flexure to make sure that the orientation is correct.
  - There is no small bowel underneath the mesentery of the left colon. In addition, if that is left in place after the anastomosis without correction, this will lead to an internal hernia and small bowel obstruction.
- The operator should hold the anvil from the depression just below the wide plastic part and never directly on the metal part with a laparoscopic Babcock forceps, and direct it toward the spike of the stapler and join the two parts. A click should be felt at that point. Occasionally, the operator would need to apply very gentle pressure from the back of the anvil to push it toward the spike.
- Once that step is done, make sure again that the orientation is correct by following the colon toward the splenic flexure, and checking the cut edge of the mesentery. Still at this point, you can change the position of the colon and change the direction of the colon. If all is okay, then the second assistant can now turn the knob to completely close the stapler (Figure 9-32). Then, the safety is released and the stapler should be fired using two hands. After that is done, the stapler is removed gently from the anal canal in an arc-like movement.
- A leak test can be done by using a flexible sigmoidoscopy, a rigid sigmoidoscopy, or even with the bulb syringe. Our preference is to use the flexible sigmoidoscopy. The operator should

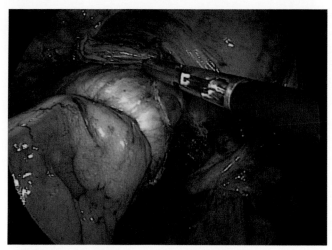

Figure 9-32. Coupling the two parts of the stapler: the anvil and the spike.

use the suction irrigation device to fill the pelvis with water. Decreasing the Trendelenburg position will help to keep the water in the pelvis, but make sure that the small bowel does not slide to the pelvis. Place an atraumatic grasper over the left colon proximal to the anastomosis, while the second assistant inserts the flexible sigmoidoscope (Figure 9-33).

- The advantages of using the flexible sigmoidoscopy includes the ability to inspect the anastomosis, and the mucosa proximal to the staple line, and to check on the completeness of the circular staple line and making sure there is no bleeding from the staple line, and if there is any bleeding, necessary intervention can be done at that time.

- Insulate the rectum to test the anastomosis. If there is no leak, then the air should be evacuated.

- At that point, all the water should be suctioned from the pelvis. Hemostasis should be checked.

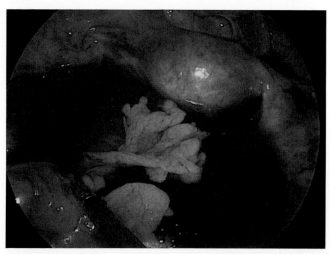

Figure 9-33. Applying gentle pressure on the left colon just proximal to the anastomosis to do the leak test.

- If there is a positive air leak:
  - ○ The best course of action is to redo the anastomosis, especially if the air-leak is significant or the site of leak is not easily accessible.
  - ○ However, if the leak is small, or can be seen easily anteriorly, then place a simple suture to close the defect, and redo the leak test to ensure that it is negative. Consider diverting the patient in that situation. Also, consider leaving a drain in the pelvis.

Stoma Creation

- Adjust the position of the bed to a maximum Trendelenburg position, with the right side up. Identify the cecum and the terminal ileum. Run the bowel proximally up to around 30 cm proximal to the ileocecal valve. Hold the mesentery just as close to the bowel as possible with an atraumatic locking grasper and exteriorize it via the midline incision, the loop is exteriorized and an umbilical tape passed right underneath the loop. The stoma opening in the pre-marked stoma site is created and the loop exteriorized.
- At this point, the small bowel can act help to close that defect and pneumoperitoneum can be established again.
- Check the orientation of the bowel, and make sure that there is no twist in the mesentery. Assess the location of the proximal and distal limbs of the stoma.
- After that is done, remove all the trocars under direct supervision.
- Evacuate the pneumoperitoneum, and then remove the Hasson trocar.
- Close all the wounds, cover them, and then mature the stoma in a Brooke fashion.

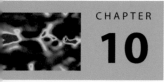

10

Laparoscopic Hartmann's Reversal

Hartmann's procedure is an eponymous procedure named after Professor Henri Hartmann. It was first described for sigmoid cancer and consisted of a segmental resection of the sigmoid colon, closure of the rectal stump, and end colostomy using the distal descending colon. Now the operation is done in cases where a segmental resection of the left/sigmoid colon is needed and it is too risky to perform a primary anastomosis. Common indications include perforated sigmoid colon (due to diverticulitis, stercoral perforation, trauma, etc.), cases of colon obstruction due to left/sigmoid colon, or upper rectal lesions. It can be safely performed laparoscopically or open. However, the majority of these cases are done using the open approach due to several factors: dilated bowel loops can make the laparoscopic approach much more difficult due to lack of working space, these patients tend to be acutely ill needing the surgery to be expeditious, and unstable patients may also have a difficult time tolerating pneumoperitoneum. Additionally, the open approach makes a thorough washout easier to perform and saves time.

Hartman's reversal after an abdominal catastrophe is challenging due to many factors. First, there will be lots of adhesions, which will make the initial laparoscopic access difficult, and occasionally unsafe. Second, dissection of the rectal stump can be challenging.

The timing of the operation is important. It is advisable that the decision to reverse the stoma after a major catastrophe in the abdomen is at least 6 months to 1 year, preferably the latter. This would allow more time for the adhesions to soften and make it more likely to complete the surgery in a minimally invasive fashion. The operation consists of multiple steps:

- Colostomy takedown/accessing the abdomen and preparing the left colon.
- Lysis of adhesions.
- Mobilization of the left colon.
- Mobilization and possible transection of the rectum.
- Creation of colorectal anastomosis.
- Flexible sigmoidoscopy to test the anastomosis.
- Assess for the need of temporary diversion.

Preoperative Considerations

Ureteral Stents

Ureteral stents placement should be considered preoperatively, to facilitate the identification of the both ureters, especially if the index surgery was difficult, if the patient has a history of ureteral injury, or if the rectal stump is short. In such cases, the scarring can be dense and the rectal dissection may be more extensive, and the ureters may be medialized due to the previous operation.

Preoperative Imaging

A pouchogram of the rectal stump can help in defining the length of the remaining rectum and its anatomy. If the patient has had a recent colonoscopy with visualization of the rectum and assessment of its length then no preoperative imaging is necessary. Most often these patients have imaging secondary to their primary pathology, namely cancer, and these can be used in preoperative planning, especially judging the need for takedown of the splenic flexure.

If the index operation was done for cancer, then prior to the operation, re-staging of the patient is necessary to make sure that there is no metastasis.

Rectal Enemas

It's advisable to prepare the rectal stump the night before and the day of surgery with a fleet enema. This will clear the rectum, and evacuate any remnant stool. This would prevent any issues during the insertion of the circular stapler. Occasionally, due to the long diversion, stool might become hard, and might cause an issue with advancing the circular stapler to the end of the rectal stump. We also perform irrigation of the rectal stump on the operating table on the day of surgery with dilute Betadine solution.

Preoperative Endoscopy

If the patient has not had a recent colonoscopy then complete evaluation of the colon prior to reversal of the Hartmann is necessary. It is important that the rectal stump is visualized as well during such a procedure. Flexible endoscopy to the rectal stump will help to estimate the length of the rectal stump and will rule out any pathology in the rectal stump such as polyps or cancer. It is common to see diversion proctitis in the form of friable and edematous mucosa with contact bleeding. It is safe to ignore this in a patient who does not have prior history of rectal disease.

Preparation of the Abdomen

- Prior to prepping the abdomen, consider closing the stoma opening with a 2-0 Vicryl suture to prevent any contamination to the field.
- The abdomen is prepped and draped per standard. However, two points should be considered:
  - First, when prepping the stoma and skin around the stoma, Povidone-Iodine prep should be used instead of Chlorhexidine. The rest of the abdomen can be prepped by Chlorhexidine prep.
  - Second, after the prep is done as discussed, place a folded surgical gauze sponge on top of the stoma to cover it, and while holding the surgical gauze sponge, place a clear waterproof dressing (e.g., Tegaderm/Ioban) on top to isolate the stoma from the abdomen and prevent any leakage of stool to the wound.

Port Sites

In Hartman's reversal, port site placement should be very flexible depending on the situation, the degree of intra-abdominal adhesions, and old scars.

However, our preference is the Alexis Laparoscopic System with Kii® Fios® First Entry through the Stoma site, with two 5-mm trocars (Figure 10-1).

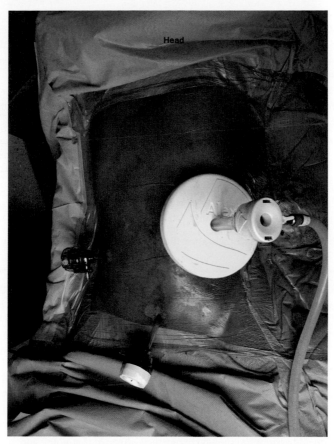

Figure 10-1. The Alexis Laparoscopic System with laparoscopic cap is used at the stoma site after the colostomy is taken down, with two 5-mm ports, in the RLQ, and suprapubic area.

Steps of the Operation

Access the Abdominal Cavity/Stoma Takedown and Preparation of the Descending Colon

- In cases where the index operation was a done for benign disease, we start the case by colostomy takedown. However, in cases where the index operation was done for cancer, then consider accessing the abdomen from the left upper quadrant (LUQ) or midline, if appropriate, and general exploration of the abdominal cavity is performed, and intraperitoneal carcinomatosis is ruled out prior to colostomy closure. Moreover, keeping the colostomy takedown to a later stage in the operation should be considered as well if there is anticipation of technical difficulties, which could lead to the inability to complete the operation. In this case, access the abdomen from a different location, such as the supraumbilical area or LUQ, using the cutdown technique.

- An incision is made at the mucocutaneous junction at the site of the prior colostomy, and this is taken down through the abdominal fat up to the level of the fascia, and careful dissection is carried out to separate the colon circumferentially from the fascia. After the colostomy is completely taken down, the colon, which was part of the stoma, is resected between a Kocher clamp and a bowel clamp.
- It is very important to make sure that the blood supply is adequate in the descending colon before creating the purse string and returning the bowel to the abdomen. This can be done using the following methods when the colon is grossly viable (pink, apparently well perfused):
  - ○ Look for visible pulsation in the small pericolonic blood vessels, making the colonic serosa moist with saline can sometimes help reflect light while observing the mesenteric aspect of the bowel wall.
  - ○ While ligating the mesocolon close to the colon wall, use Metzenbaum scissors to divide the mesentery while having a hemostat ready to clamp the mesocolon after division. If there is bleeding, then it is reassuring that the blood supply is adequate.
  - ○ Another method of checking is using fluorescence imaging to visualize the perfusion.

⚠ Caution: Keep in mind while you mobilize the left colon that it may be necessary to divide more mesocolon to get enough mobility of the left colon to allow it to reach to the pelvis. However, if that is done, the distal part of the left colon should be checked again to make sure there is no compromise in the blood supply.

- A 2-0 Prolene suture is used to create purse string in the proximal bowel, and the anvil of the circular stapler is placed, and secured with the purse sting. At this point, it is prudent to save as much colon as feasible especially in cases where colon length could be a limiting factor in restoring intestinal continuity. The bowel is returned back to the abdominal cavity.
- The surgeon and assistant(s) should change their gloves at that point, and all the instruments that were used for the stoma should not be used again to decrease the incidence of superficial surgical site infection.
- Now, there are two options:
  - ○ Our preference is to use an Alexis Laparoscopic System with Kii® Fios® First Entry and laparoscopic cap, to establish pneumoperitoneum. This is an easy and quick way to access the abdomen, establish pneumoperitoneum, and plan the sites of the other trocars. If the wound protector will be used without the laparoscopic cap, then the assistant holds the Hassan trocar and places it inside the wound protector, and the surgeon twists the wound protector around itself. The assistant can use a 0-silk suture or an umbilical tape to tie around the Hassan trocar. This will create a tight seal. A wet lap is placed in the wound, and wrapped around the Hassan trocar, and then the wound protector is turned in the usual fashion until it reaches the level of the skin.
  - ○ Alternatively, close the stoma site using 0-PDS sutures in a figure of eight fashion to close the defect, and tie them except for two stitches that are at the most cephalad part of the wound. The Hasson trocar is inserted through it, and the sutures, are tied around it.
  - ○ Advantage: One big advantage of using this technique is accessing the abdomen relatively safely, and avoiding the complications of midline entry especially if the patient has had a laparotomy before, where adhesions are expected to be in the midline of the incision, and may lead to complications during accessing the abdomen.

- Two 5-mm trocars are inserted under direct supervision in the right lower quadrant (RLQ) and the suprapubic area.

- This configuration can vary significantly depending on the distribution of the adhesions to the abdominal wall, which may hinder the placement of the 5-mm trocars in the suprapubic area and RLQ right away. In case of adhesions to the abdominal wall, add another 5-mm trocar in the area of the abdomen that is clear of adhesions to help with lysis of adhesions. After the adhesions are lysed and a clear window is created, now it's safe to place the 5-mm trocars in the desired location—typically the right side and the suprapubic area.

- A single incision laparoscopic port is placed in the colostomy site. A 5-mm supraumbilical port site is placed. A 5-mm, 30° camera is used via this port and the single incision port is used for remainder of the case including mobilization of the left colon, splenic flexure, and rectal stump mobilization, etc.

Lysis of Adhesions (Figures 10-2 to 10-4)

- The purpose of this step is to take down the adhesions in the midline, lower abdomen, and the right abdomen in order to place the ports safely and perform the operation. It's important to know that not every single adhesion needs to be taken down.

- This should be done sharply using laparoscopic scissors.

- To establish this task, extra port placement should be considered to accomplish this. For example. The initial access site could be the colostomy site or a cutdown in the LUQ. In that case, 5-mm ports can be placed in the left abdomen, under direct supervision, to lyse adhesions in the midline, and then the right abdomen, which allow placement of trocars in the right abdomen in order to do the pelvic dissection, and the mobilization of the left colon.

- Consider using a 5-mm camera, if needed, to help with the lysis of adhesions, by using the 5 mm ports that was placed in the left abdomen.

- Take down the adhesions using laparoscopic scissors. Very gentle blunt dissection can be used just to create a plane for dissection. Avoid using any energy source since the heat transmission can cause unrecognized bowel injury.

Abdominal Operations

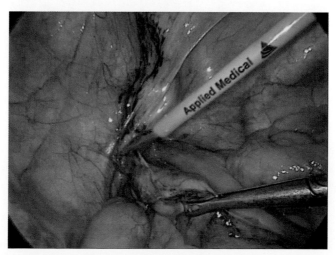

Figure 10-2. Lysis of adhesions between the small bowel and the pelvis.

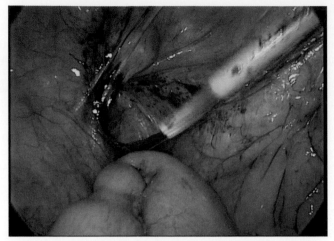

Figure 10-3. Clearing all small bowel loops from the pelvis by sharp lysis of adhesions.

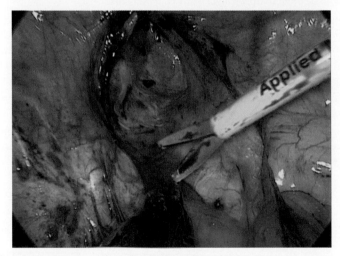

Figure 10-4. The pelvis is cleared now from the small bowel.

Mobilization of the Left Colon (Figures 10-5 to 10-8)

- The patient should be placed in the Trendelenburg position with the left side up.

- The anvil should be identified, and then the left colon should be mobilized lateral to medial. The colon is grasped from the epiploica, and pulled medially, and then the dissection starts from that level just medial to the white line of Toldt.

- The dissection continues until the splenic flexure is taken down completely. Repositioning the bed to reverse Trendelenburg position can help with the flexure takedown. Enter the lesser sac, and divide the omentum off the transverse colon. After that, the reach to the upper rectum is checked.

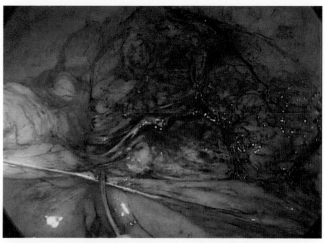

Figure 10-5. Mobilizing the left colon and division of the attachments to the retroperitoneum and Gerota's fascia.

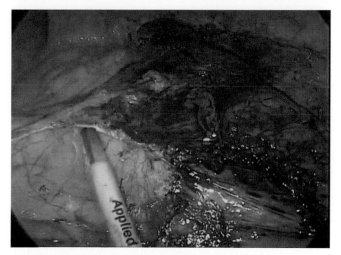

Figure 10-6. Continuing the lateral mobilization by separating the left colon from Gerota's fascia.

Mobilization and Possible Transection of the Rectum

- Now, the dissection of the rectal stump starts. If there are any small bowel loops stuck to the pelvis, lysis of adhesions is performed to remove these loops of bowel from the pelvis.
- If there is any difficulty with identification of the rectal stump, rectal sizers can be placed to identify the stump, and know its course. Alternatively, flexible sigmoidoscopy can be placed and this would help with the identification of the stump.
- Identify the left ureter to avoid injury.
- Start mobilizing the rectal stump by holding the staple line and pull it to the right side, and start dividing the left pararectal sulcus. Extreme care is taken not to injure the left ureter. Then dissection starts on the right pararectal sulcus in the same manner. Posterior dissection in the TME plane is started and the dissection continues until it's felt that the stump is mobilized.

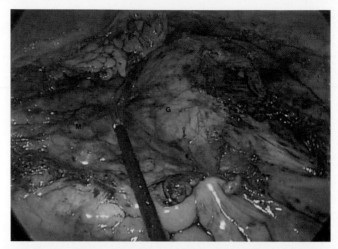

Figure 10-7. The mesentery of the left colon (M) is completely dissected off Gerota's fascia (G).

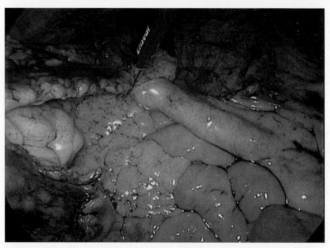

Figure 10-8. Division of the mesentery of the left colon to reach to the pelvis. Notice that this step could lead to ischemia of the left colon if the distal part of the left colon is de-vascularized.

- The dissection of the rectum should be limited. The goal of the rectal mobilization is it to mobilize just enough in order to place the circular stapler and restore the gastrointestinal continuity.
- One way to assess if the dissection is enough is to place the rectal sizer, and if it reaches up to the staple line, then the circular stapler can be placed to create the anastomosis.
- One of the pitfalls in this case is difficulty with inserting the circular stapler. Please refer to Chapter 19, titled "Misadventure with Stapling Devices" for further details.

Creation of Colorectal Anastomosis

- Prior to making the anastomosis, a leak test of the rectal stump is performed to make sure there is no leak from the staple line from the rectal stump.

- In case there is a leak, or if the stapler cannot be advanced to the end of the staple line, re-resection of the rectal stump is needed. This is performed up to the level where the circular stapler can reach. End-to-end anastomosis is performed. Alternatively, an end-to-side anastomosis can be performed, where the spike of the circular stapler is introduced via the anterior wall of the rectal stump if it was not able to reach to the end of the staple line.

Flexible Sigmoidoscopy to Test the Anastomosis

A leak test is performed using flexible sigmoidoscopy. In addition to that, flexible sigmoidoscopy will aid to visualize the anastomosis, make sure that there is no active bleeding from the staple line, and assess the color of the mucosa of the colon.

Assess for the Need of Temporary Diversion

Rarely if ever, proximal diversion will be needed in these cases.

Alternative Technique*

- Start with accessing the abdomen through a cut-down technique in the LUQ or the RUQ. Place the ports under direct super vision. After the adhesiolysis is accomplished, and after confirming that the reversal can be done, the anvil is placed through the stoma and pushed inside the lumen of the bowel where it can laparoscopically be seen.

- A suture should be placed at the opening in the spike of the anvil, so it can be pulled and manipulated laparoscopically.

- An endo GIA stapler is used to divide the stoma close to the abdominal wall making sure that the anvil is below the staple line. The take down of the remaining part of the colostomy is done at the end of the case.

- A colotomy is made in the bowel just beside the staple line. A fishing technique is applied using the hook to "fish for the suture" that was attached at the end of the spike. Once that is identified, it is pulled through. The spike of the anvil should be removed.

- An Endoloop is used to create a tight seal around the anvil.

- Then, a colorectal anastomosis and leak test is performed as usual.

- After the laparoscopic part is done, and the incisions are closed, colostomy takedown is performed, and then fascia and skin are closed in a standard fashion.

*Reference: https://www.websurg.com/doi/lt03enleroy013/

Abdominal Operations

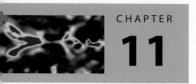

Abdominoperineal Resection

Abdominoperineal resection (APR) refers to the removal of a portion of the left colon, the entire rectum and anus, and creation of an end colostomy. It should be considered when the tumor is invading the anal canal, sphincter complex, or the pelvic floor; if the surgeon can't get a negative distal-free resection margin in very low rectal tumors; if the patient has fecal incontinence preoperatively; or patient preference. The initial steps of the operation are the same as laparoscopic low anterior resection (LAR) so, in some ways, this chapter is a continuation of the LAR chapter.

Preoperative Considerations

Ureteral Stents

In general, ureteral stent placement is preferable in APR. Placing bilateral stents will allow the surgeon to identify the ureters during the pelvic part of the operation. This is important especially if the tumor is bulky and if there is extensive fibrosis in the tissues due to radiation. Occasionally, even with the stents, it's difficult to identify, and extreme care should be exercised during the pelvic dissection.

Imaging

Review the pelvic magnetic resonance imaging (MRI) of the patient carefully, because it will provide you with a road map to the operation. There are many useful pieces of information that you need to get from the MRI before you start, which includes:

- Location of tumor.
- T stage of tumor.
- Lymph nodal enlargement (N staging).
- Distance of tumor from anorectal ring/sphincter complex.
- Involvement of surrounding organs (prostate, seminal vesicles, bladder, ureter, uterus, vagina) or anal sphincters complex.
- Relationship of tumor to the line joining the sacral promontory to symphysis pubis. Any tumor below this line is in the true pelvis. Such tumors should be considered for preoperative chemoradiation treatment if they are T3 or higher or have node-positive disease.

Margins

In all cancer cases, adequate margins are paramount. For upper rectal cancer, getting adequate margins is not difficult and we aim for a 3–5-cm margin. In mid-to-low rectal cancers, 1–2 cm of negative margin should be ideal but 0.5–1-cm margins are acceptable. However, for sphincter preservation, we perform intraoperative frozen section and aim for negative margins. If the tumor is very low, and a negative margin cannot be achieved, APR should be done. In addition, during the resection of the mesentery, the IMA should be divided at its origin. This maximizes adequate lymph node harvest. Prior to starting the case, carrying out a digital rectal examination is important because this helps make an accurate final clinical assessment of how low the tumor is, especially because the last clinical exam may have been weeks prior to the surgery. In female patients with anterior tumors, we also do a vaginal exam to rule out involvement of the posterior vaginal wall.

Rectal Washout

We routinely perform rectal washout in all left-sided and rectal cancer cases. A size 30-French red rubber catheter, or alternatively, a Foley catheter, is inserted in the rectum, and then diluted iodine is instilled in the rectum. While instilling the iodine, the catheter should be elevated above the level of the bed, and then lowered down to evacuate the rectum.

Steps to All Operations

All the initial steps are the same as described in the laparoscopic LAR chapter. One important difference is the left colon and splenic flexure mobilization. In APR, the left colon is mobilized enough to allow for creation of left sided colostomy. Most of the time, splenic flexure mobilization is not required, unless the left colon is short or the patient is obese, then splenic flexure mobilization is needed to allow for creation of the colostomy without tension.

The pelvic dissection should be continued laparoscopically to the level of the levator muscle complex. At this level, the laparoscopic dissection should be stopped and the perineal part should be started. A common pitfall is that the surgeon continues the dissection from the abdominal approach, toward the anorectum. This will lead, inadvertently, to thinning of the distal part of the rectum leading to the formation of a "waist" in the specimen instead of the ideal cylindrical APR specimen

The perineal part can be done concomitantly with the patient in high lithotomy position if there are two surgical teams or consequently after finishing the abdominal part if there is only a single surgical team or if the surgeon prefers to prone the patient for the perineal part of the case. Most commonly, the perineal part is done in the lithotomy position, with the legs placed high on yellow fins stirrups to allow maximal exposure. Of note, during the beginning of the case, the legs should be low to prevent any interference with the surgeon during the abdominal part of the operation, and later on during the case, the legs can be adjusted.

Although the prone jackknife position can give superior view of the anatomy, and allow the assistant to assist the surgeon more easily, it requires flipping the patient, and redraping. In addition, if the dissection was not complete from the abdominal part, it will be a problem because there is no access to the abdomen in that position, to help the surgeon to finish the perineal part. The prone position is useful in certain subset of patients and we use it for obese male patients when the lithotomy position may not provide excellent access to the perineum. However, this same exact reason (i.e., high body mass index) can be hazardous as well during flipping the patient in the prone jackknife position. So careful communication with the anesthetist and the operating room (OR) team should be done prior to starting the operation.

When doing the perineal portion in high lithotomy position, the patient has to be low enough on the OR table to facilitate the dissection. A gel pad/rolled blankets can be positioned at the beginning of the case underneath the sacrum and coccyx. This will elevate the pelvis and it will facilitate the exposure during the perineal part.

The anus can be sutured closed with a purse string suture to prevent any soilage. If digital access is needed during the case to palpate the coccyx or prostate, then this suture can be removed and two Allis clamps can be used to close the anus and facilitate retraction.

The surgeon should wear a headlight, to allow for optimal visualization.

A diamond-shaped incision (which can be modified to a circle; see Figure 11-1) is made, taking into consideration the key landmarks, which are the coccyx posteriorly, ischial tuberosities in both sides, and the perineal body anteriorly. The dissection should be started posteriorly, which is considered the safest. A Lone Star retractor system is utilized for better exposure (Figure 11-2). Alternatively, multiple sutures can be used to efface the anorectal area, and can mimic the effects of the Lone Star. The surgeon should identify the coccyx, and then the dissection should start in front of the coccyx until the anococcygeal ligament is divided. This is a key step in the perineal dissection. In thin people, this step is easy, but care should be exercised in obese patients when the coccyx is hard to feel, and the dissection plane can easily go posterior to the coccyx. To avoid that, constant assessment of the coccyx is paramount, and the direction of the dissection should be adjusted accordingly. After the pelvic cavity is entered from the posterior plane of dissection, then the surgeon can sweep their finger in both directions; right and left, and hook the levator complex muscles, and then the lateral dissection should start, by dividing these muscles as lateral as possible. LigaSure can be used to ensure adequate hemostasis.

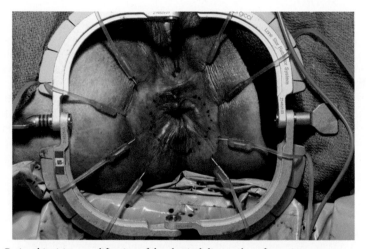

Figure 11-1. Perineal incision, modification of the classical diamond configuration.

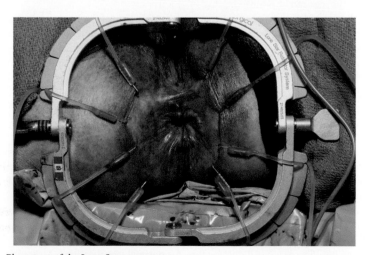

Figure 11-2. Placement of the Lone Star retractor.

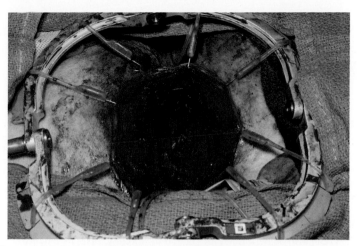

Figure 11-3. Perineal defect after specimen extraction with the first layer of sutures in place.

During this time, multiple Allis clamps can be placed on the anus, to be used as retractor to pull the specimen out, and direct it to any direction, to facilitate the dissection, a pediatric Deaver retractor can be used by the assistant to provide countertraction. After the lateral dissection is done on both sides, then the dissection should be continued from the sides to the anterior plane with care. The specimen can be extracted posteriorly after the lateral and posterior dissection is complete. The staple line is held by the operator from the abdomen and delivered to the operator in the perineum who can hold it with a Babcock and flip the rectum outward and "deliver" the specimen. The last part of the dissection is the anterior plane, which is usually the most challenging one. Anteriorly in males, the urethra can be injured especially if the tumor is located anteriorly, and wider margins anteriorly are required. Palpating for the Foley catheter can be helpful to identify if the plane of the dissection is close to the urethra or not. In females, the vagina is at risk of injury, and a clean gloved finger can be inserted in the vagina to help identify the wall of the vagina and help with the anterior dissection.

Furthermore, the purse string suture that was used to close the anus at the beginning to avoid spillage can be opened, and an index finger can be inserted to help identify the anterior plane. This will facilitate identifying the area of dissection anteriorly. While retracting the specimen outward, the dissection should be continued anteriorly, layer by layer, going through the superficial perineal muscle, and developing the plane between the rectum and prostate/vagina. The dissection is continued until the specimen is completely separated. Irrigation of the pelvis is performed to make sure the hemostasis is adequate, and then a drain is placed from the abdomen to the pelvis. The perineal wound is closed in layers by absorbable sutures (Figure 11-3), and a perineal drain can also be placed in select patients. Patients who have a large perineal defect after an APR may need perineal reconstruction with a muscle flap such as a vertical rectus abdominis myocutaneous (VRAM) flap; the need for this is usually apparent during preoperative assessment and the surgery should be planned accordingly.

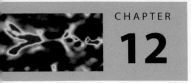

Laparoscopic Total Abdominal Colectomy

Laparoscopic total abdominal colectomy (TAC) entails the removal of the entire colon up to the top of the rectum. Intestinal continuity may be restored in the form of ileorectal anastomosis or an end ileostomy may be fashioned depending on the indication for surgery, patient's general condition, and condition of the colon and the rectum. TAC is the procedure of choice for patients who are acutely ill from pancolitis due to ulcerative colitis, Crohn's disease, or *Clostridium difficile* colitis; for patients who have severe colonic bleeding without accurate preoperative localization or obstructing left colon cancer with evidence of perforation; or ischemia in the right colon. In these situations, it is performed urgently. Electively, TAC can also be performed for colonic dysmotility, cases of synchronous colon cancer, selected patients with inflammatory bowel disease, and colon polyposis syndrome patients who are candidates for ileorectal anastomosis.

This operative description is for chronic ulcerative colitis, or Stage I procedure.

Preoperative Considerations

Steroids

Patients with chronic ulcerative colitis are most likely on chronic steroids. Patients who are taking steroids preoperatively should be given a stress dose of Hydrocortisone 50–100 mg IV in the perioperative area before surgery. Postoperatively, the steroids should be weaned depending on the preoperative dose, and the duration of use.

Stoma Marking

Preoperative marking with the enterostomal nurse is essential to ensure the best position for a planned stoma, and to avoid issues related to inappropriate positioning.

Positioning

Use the modified lithotomy position.

Port Sites

Four Ports Diamond-Shaped Configuration (Figure 12-1)

- This configuration will allow you to do the total abdominal colectomy and work in all the abdominal quadrants.
- A supraumbilical port (12 mm) is used for the camera.
- Two 5-mm ports are placed in the suprapubic area and the left lower quadrant (LLQ).
- Right lower quadrant (RLQ) port: This port can be placed through the planned stoma site, if appropriate. Make a circular incision at the planned stoma site. Deepen the incision and continue with the dissection around the skin and subcutaneous fat

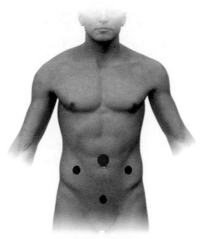

Figure 12-1. Four ports diamond-shaped configuration. The red circle represents a 12-mm site for the camera, and the blue circles are 5-mm ports.

Abdominal Operations

in a cylindrical shape until the fascia is reached. Then the fat can be amputated and discarded. Now, the fascia should be visible. This technique can be used if the abdominal wall is thick, and this would help with delivering the stoma at the end of the case and mature it. If the abdominal wall is thin, then after making the circular skin incision, place the 12-mm trocar in the usual fashion. This incision will not need to be closed, since it will be the future stoma site and this by default will be enlarged. The caveat is that the site of this trocar may not be the usual typical location of the port, since it has to be adjusted for the stoma site. If the site for ostomy marked by the stoma nurse is not ideal for port placement then it is best not to use it. Placing a 5-mm port at the desired location for smooth conduct of the operation is much better than compromising on the site of the port in order to use the proposed ostomy site.

For Left Colon and Sigmoid Mobilization

- Four ports can be used; three 5-mm trocars are placed in the RLQ, LLQ, and the suprapubic area, and a 12-mm trocar in the supraumbilical area.
- Suprapubic port: This port can be used during the mobilization of the left colon, and sigmoid colon. Laparoscopic scissors, hook, or a vessel-sealing device can be used. Also, this port can be utilized during splenic flexure mobilization using an atraumatic grasper, to expose, and use an energy source in the LLQ port. In obese patients, long instrument may be needed if you are utilizing the suprapubic port to retract and help with splenic flexure mobilization.
- To retract the colon, an atraumatic grasper can be utilized through either the suprapubic port, or the RLQ port, and the LLQ port can be used to mobilize the splenic flexure and distal transverse colon using an energy device.
- LLQ port: This port can be used during mobilization of the splenic flexure and the distal transverse colon. A dissecting instrument such as a laparoscopic hook, scissors, or an energy source can be used through this port to take down the splenic flexure.

For Right Colon Mobilization

- The LLQ port can used to retract the colon and expose the white line of Toldt while laparoscopic scissors can be used through the suprapubic port to mobilize the right colon. if you do the reverse, by holding the laparoscopic scissors or energy source with your right hand through the LLQ, and use the suprapubic port for retraction, there will be crossing of the instruments inside the abdomen which is not ideal but allows the right-handed surgeon to control the scissors with their dominant hand. for

- In high–BMI patients, a left upper quadrant (LUQ) 5-mm port can be placed to help with the flexure takedown. At that point, the surgeon can use both the LUQ and LLQ ports.

Four Ports Plus Two Additional Ports

- One or two additional ports can be used in this case, in the right upper quadrant (RUQ) and LUQ. They can be useful in high-BMI patients, where the usual instruments will not be able to reach the upper abdomen, or in high splenic flexure (Figure 12-2).

Steps of the Operation

In patients with chronic ulcerative colitis, lateral-to-medial mobilization is preferred, because high ligation of the vessels is not critical in this operation. We start the procedure from the left side but one can decide to start from the right side. The operation involves the following steps:

1. Abdominal exploration.
2. Mobilization of the left colon.
3. Division of the bowel distally.
4. Division of the mesentery of the sigmoid colon and descending colon.
5. Splenic flexure mobilization.
6. Mobilization of the right colon.
7. Mobilizing the remaining transverse colon and division of the remaining mesentery of the transverse colon.
8. Exteriorization of the specimen.
9. Division of the terminal ileum and creation of stoma/anastomosis and closure.

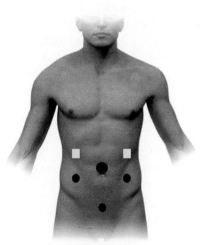

Figure 12-2. Four ports plus two additional ports. The red circle represents a 12-mm site for the camera, and the blue circles are 5-mm ports, and the yellow squares represent extra two additional ports that can be used as well.

Abdominal Exploration

Explore the abdominal cavity for ascites, carcinomatosis, or unexpected liver lesions, especially if the indication for surgery in chronic ulcerative colitis is cancer.

Mobilization of the Left Colon

- Both the surgeon and the assistant stand on the patient's right side with the monitor across the table.
- Position the operating room bed in the Trendelenburg position, and left side up.
- Bring all the small intestine out of the pelvis.
- Reflect the omentum above the transverse colon.
- Using an atraumatic grasper through the RLQ port, hold the fat at the level of the sigmoid colon at the pelvic brim and pull it medially and upward toward the ceiling. Start by using laparoscopic scissors with cautery or any vessel-sealing device, such as LigaSure, through the suprapubic port to mobilize the sigmoid colon. Divide the lateral attachments just medial to the white line of Toldt. This plane of dissection is bloodless if one stays in the correct plane. A lot of the mobilization can be accomplished by gentle "pushing and pulling" with the bowel grasper or laparoscopic scissors once the surgeon is in the correct plane. Continue with this dissection cephalad toward the descending colon (Figures 12-3 to 12-7).
- Take it layer by layer until you reflect the sigmoid colon and its mesentery off the sidewall, the retroperitoneal attachments, and Gerota's fascia.
- Identify the left ureter. It can be found at the base of the sigmoid fossa.

⚠ Pitfalls: In very thin patients, the initial dissection can sometimes be difficult because the lack of fat makes it difficult to identify the correct plane. One has to be careful not to dissect lateral to Gerota's fascia.

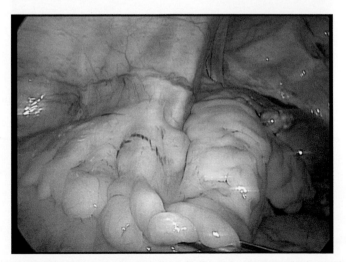

Figure 12-3. Starting the dissection from the pelvic brim, by retracting the sigmoid colon medially and starting the lateral-to-medial dissection.

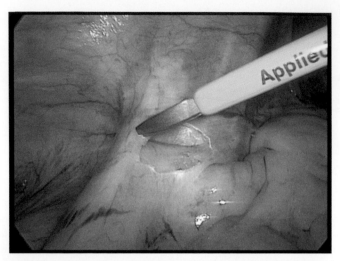

Figure 12-4. Starting the lateral dissection using laparoscopic scissors connected to electrocautery. Alternatively, any energy device can be used.

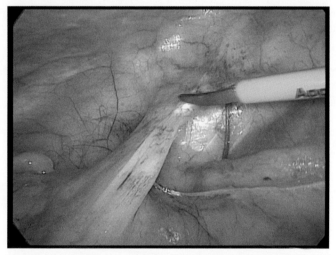

Figure 12-5. Lateral dissection should be just medial to the white line of Toldt. Notice the difference in the colon between the mesentery of the colon and the retroperitoneum.

⚠ Pitfalls: In thin patients, the mesocolon has very little fat and so it's easy to cause a defect in the mesocolon (Figures 12-8 and 12-9). This can lead to thermal injury to the underlying small bowel leading to a missed enterotomy.

Division of the Bowel Distally

- It is ergonomically best for the surgeon to remain on the right side of the patient. The assistant moves to the left side of the patient and the monitor is moved in between the legs.

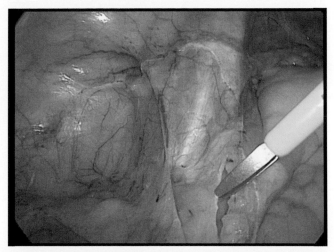

Figure 12-6. Taking the lateral attachments one layer at a time, making sure to adjust the retraction with the left hand for adequate exposure.

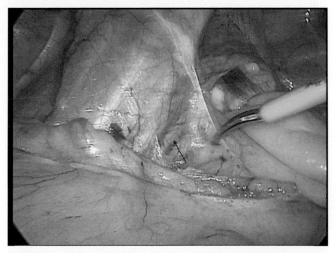

Figure 12-7. Continue with the lateral dissection toward the pelvis. Notice that the dissection started after the site of the ureter was identified, and made sure that the dissection area is away from the ureter.

- Determine the area of distal resection. As a rule, this should be at the top of the rectum. The exception would be cases where there is severe disease of the rectum and one plans to bring up the distal sigmoid as a mucus fistula; in such cases, the stump is left longer so that it can reach the skin level.

- Continue with the dissection toward the pelvis, along the left pararectal sulcus. Prior to doing this, identify the left ureter again, and make sure it's away from the dissection area.

- Hold the distal sigmoid colon using atraumatic grasper and pull it medially toward the midline using the RLQ port, and use laparoscopic scissors in the suprapubic port to dissect the sigmoid from the left pelvic sidewall until just below the area of distal resection. The level of resection should be at the top of the rectum. Dissecting the rectum distally is unnecessary and should be avoided.

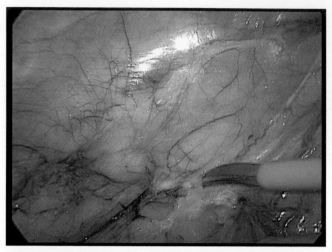

Figure 12-8. Notice here that the dissection plane was too medial, and led to the creation of a hole in the mesentery of the colon. Notice that the small bowel that can be seen from that defect.

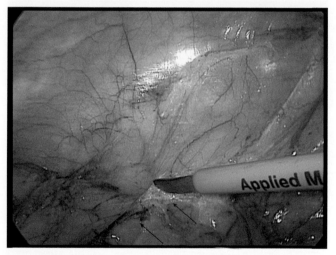

Figure 12-9. Restoring the correct dissecting plane (red arrow), just a little bit lateral to the mesenteric defect that was created (blue arrow).

- Using an atraumatic grasper through the RLQ port, the surgeon can hold the mesentery of the sigmoid and lift it upward, while using an energy source or laparoscopic scissors through the suprapubic port, to score the peritoneal layer over the mesentery of the sigmoid colon and then continue distally toward the intended site of resection, and then at that point, score the mesocolon perpendicular toward the rectal wall. A second assistant can help out by holding the sigmoid colon using the LLQ port, especially when the sigmoid colon mesentery is heavy and bulky.
- Division of the mesocolon should be done using any vessel-sealing device at the intended level of resection. This can be done by opening the jaw of the vessel sealing device, and placing the upper jaw in the mesorectum, just posterior to the rectal wall, and before the jaw of the energy

device is closed, pull it down gently to get off the posterior wall of the rectum to create a safe distance between the vessel sealing device and the posterior rectal wall, then activate the vessel sealing device and divide. This move will prevent any thermal injury to the posterior wall of the rectum. Continue doing this until the posterior wall of the rectum is completely cleared and a generous window is created in the mesocolon.

- The surgeon should use the RLQ port to pull the rectum to the right, exposing the left side of the rectum. The second assistant who is standing on the left side of the patient can provide countertraction to the surgeon by using an atraumatic grasper. Divide the remaining part of the mesocolon to complete the creation of the mesocolic window. Thus, the rectum is cleared circumferentially and ready for division (Figures 12-10 to 12-12).

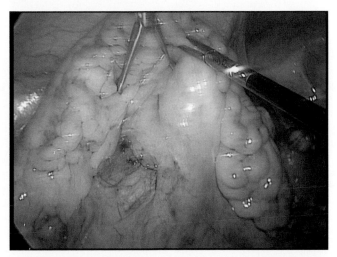

Figure 12-10. The second assistant is holding the sigmoid colon using the LLQ port to expose the medial side of the mesentery of the sigmoid colon.

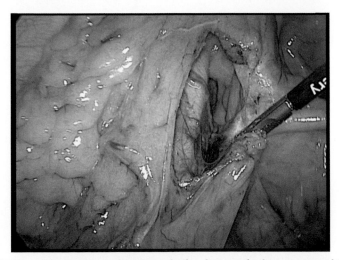

Figure 12-11. Division of the mesentery of the sigmoid colon directing the dissection toward the posterior wall of rectosigmoid.

Abdominal Operations

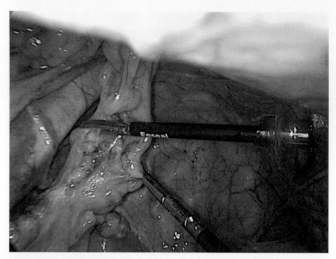

Figure 12-12. Clearing the posterior wall of the rectosigmoid colon using an energy source in preparation for stapling.

- Place the Endo GIA 60-mm stapler through the 12-mm port in the RLQ (upsize to 12 mm if a 5-mm port was placed initially or use the supraumbilical post for stapling with a 5-mm camera placed in one of the lateral ports). Reticulate the stapler so it can be perpendicular to the rectal wall as much as possible. Use the atraumatic bowel grasper through LLQ or suprapubic port to manipulate the colon and help with positioning the colon in the Endo GIA stapler. Usually, the purple load will be sufficient for the rectal wall thickness (the stapler color coding is specific to the manufacturer so best to use the stapler height for bowel anastomosis as per the specification of your local manufacturer).

- Prior to closing the stapler, try to adjust the position of the rectum in a way to have the upper rectum fully divided with one firing of the Endo GIA stapler (Figure 12-13). Optimally, the complete division will require only one firing of the Endo GIA stapler. If another

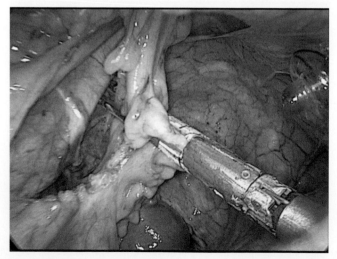

Figure 12-13. Firing a stapler across the rectosigmoid colon using an Endo GI stapler, through the RLQ port.

stapler fire is needed, then care must be taken to align the direction of the second staple line with the first one.

- Make sure there are no other structures incorporated in the stapler's jaw, namely the left ureter, and left pelvic sidewall structures.

- Fire the stapler. It is very important to be in an ergonomically comfortable position when firing the EEA stapler. It may be best to have the lower the table to a comfortable height. It is also very important not to move the stapler when squeezing the handles shut. The natural tendency is for the stapler to move forward and the surgeon should be aware of this and avoid it. The safety should be released and stapler should be fired in one smooth motion and held in place for a few seconds before releasing. After releasing, the safety should be placed back on.

Division of the Mesentery of the Sigmoid Colon and Descending Colon

- Both the surgeon and the assistant stand on the patient's right side with the monitor across the table.

- The vessel-sealing device can be used to divide the mesentery from the cut edge where the colon was divided toward the splenic flexure. Of note, during dividing the inferior mesenteric artery (IMA) pedicle, extra care should be exercised to ligate it proximally and distally prior to dividing the vessel. The IMA/superior hemorrhoidal is divided at a point of convenience that may be away from its origin, because it's not an oncological resection (Figure 12-14).

- Complete the lateral mobilization of the sigmoid colon and descending colon from its lateral attachments and from Gerota's fascia. Continue until the splenic flexure is reached (Figure 12-15).

Splenic Flexure Mobilization (Figures 12-16 to 12-20)

- At this point, the patient should be repositioned in the reverse Trendelenburg position, with the left side up.

- The surgeon can still operate from the right side of the patient; however, it would be easier for the surgeon to be in between the legs of the patient, and the monitor should be repositioned to face the surgeon. And the assistant should be standing on the right side of the patient.

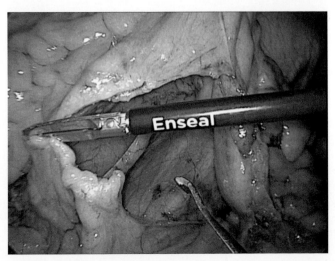

Figure 12-14. Dividing the mesentery starting from the cut edge of the mesentery toward the left colon.

Abdominal Operations

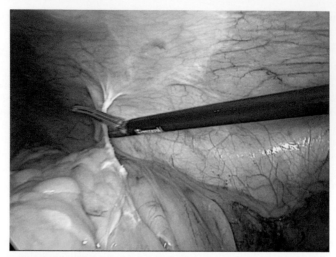

Figure 12-15. Taking down the splenic flexure attachments.

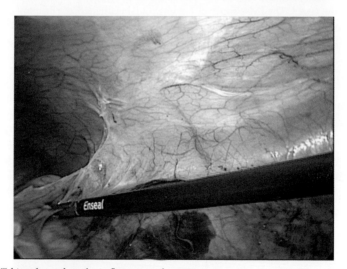

Figure 12-16. Taking down the splenic flexure attachments.

- The dissection should continue toward the splenic flexure until the splenic flexure is completely mobilized.
- The splenic flexure is attached to the spleen by multiple attachments. Mobilize the splenic flexure by gently pulling it down and medially to take the splenocolic attachment. Avoid excessive pulling; otherwise, splenic injury might occur.
- Avoid using any excessive blunt dissection in this area. If any blunt dissection is used, the direction of the dissection should be toward the colon (i.e., down and medially), not toward the spleen.
- Care should be exercised during the mobilization of the splenic flexure and during the division of the mesentery of the transverse colon, not to injure the tail of the pancreas.

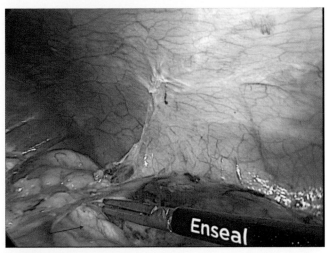

Figure 12-17. Mobilizing the splenic flexure. Notice that the pancreatic tail is very close to the dissection area, and it should be recognized and avoided.

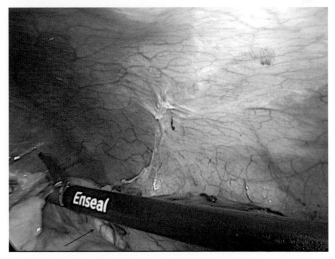

Figure 12-18. Completing the mobilization of the splenic flexure, taking care to avoid injuring the tail of the pancreas (blue arrow).

- Continue with the division of the mesentery of the transverse colon from the divided cut edge, and continue dividing the mesentery of the distal transverse colon. The division of the mesentery should continue along the transverse colon.

- Use the RLQ port and the suprapubic port to mobilize the distal transverse colon. The assistant should stand on the patient's left, and using the LLQ port, the assistant can hold the distal transverse colon using the atraumatic grasper and provide adequate exposure and traction. Left side up positioning may help in this step with the reverse Trendelenburg position.

- In high-BMI patients, or high flexure, consider adding an extra port in the RUQ to help with mobilization of the distal transverse colon. In this case, the working trocars will be the RUQ and RLQ (Figure 12-2).

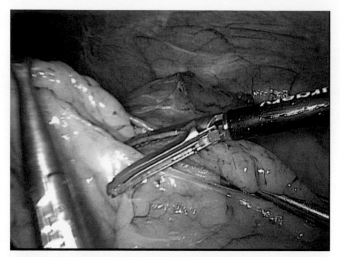

Figure 12-19. Retrograde mobilizing of the splenic flexure by entering the lesser sac and directing the dissection toward the splenic flexure.

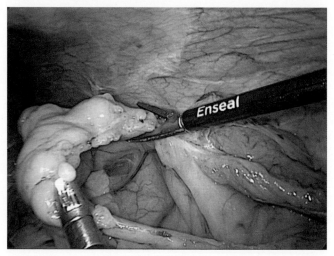

Figure 12-20. Entering the lesser sac by dividing in between the transverse colon and the stomach.

Mobilization of the Right Colon (Figures 12-21 to 12-26)

- Both the surgeon and the assistant stand on the patient's left side with the monitor across the table.
- The patient should be positioned in the Trendelenburg position, with the right side up.
- Hold the fold of Treves using an atraumatic bowel grasper using the LLQ port, and pull it medially and upward toward the abdominal wall. Through the suprapubic port, a vessel sealing device or laparoscopic scissors attached to electrocautery is used to take lateral attachment just medial to the white line of Toldt.
- The tension with the right hand should be adjusted to provide maximum traction without tearing to facilitate the dissection.

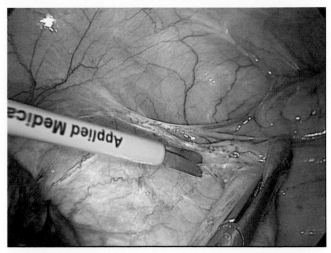

Figure 12-21. Mobilization of the terminal ileum from the right-side pelvic wall.

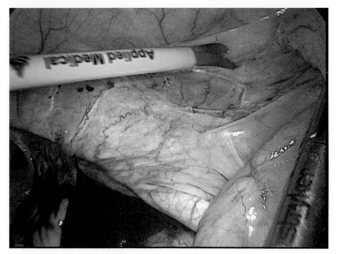

Figure 12-22. Completing the mobilization of the terminal ileum from the right-side pelvic wall.

- The dissection should continue until the hepatic flexure is reached.
- The dissection should be methodical, taking the colonic attachment one layer at a time. Returning back to the area that was initially mobilized, further dissection would be required to mobilize the ascending colon from Gerota's fascia. A rule of thumb during the dissection is that " all purple stuff goes down" to the retroperitoneum, and basically it belongs with the patient. Following this rule prevents injury to the retroperitoneal structures by keeping the surgeon in the correct plane.
- To complete the hepatic flexure take down, one can start from the middle part of the transverse colon. Repositioning the bed in the reverse Trendelenburg position allows gravity to bring down the colon and this will lead to better exposure.

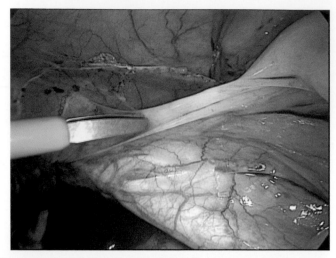

Figure 12-23. Completing the mobilization of the terminal ileum.

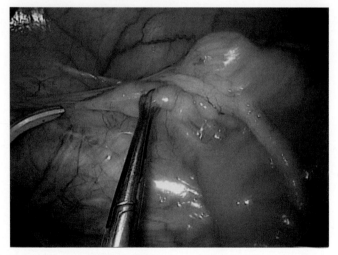

Figure 12-24. Lateral mobilization of the cecum.

- The assistant can be on the right of the patient using the RLQ port, or in between the legs using the suprapubic port. The assistant can hold the transverse colon down to provide a good exposure to the surgeon. The surgeon should stand on the patient left side, and use the suprapubic and LLQ ports to mobilize the proximal transverse colon.

- Occasionally, if the flexure is high, or in high-BMI patients, an extra port in the LUQ can help with mobilizing the proximal transverse colon and hepatic flexure. If the LUQ port is added, the surgeon can use an energy source through the LUQ port to dissect and divide the omentum and hepatic flexure attachments. With the left hand, the surgeon can use an atraumatic grasper to pull down the transverse colon and apply appropriate traction to help with the dissection.

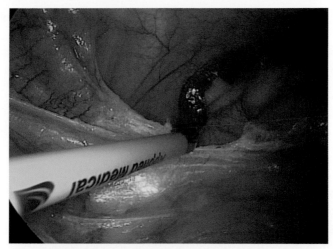

Figure 12-25. Lateral mobilization of the ascending colon one layer at a time toward the hepatic flexure.

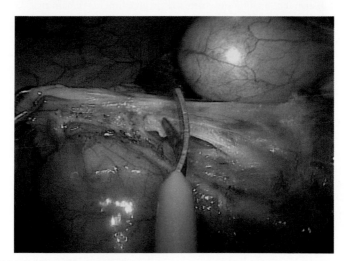

Figure 12-26. Mobilization of the hepatic flexure.

- The surgeon can start dividing between the omentum and proximal transverse colon, directing the dissection toward the hepatic flexure. The dissection should be close to the colon, but not too close to avoid any thermal injury to the colon. Start from the flimsy, transparent area in the omentum, where it will lead you to the lesser sac. The dissection should be continued gently until the hepatic flexure is reached. The assistant should follow the surgeon to provide the best exposure, and adjust the traction accordingly.

- When the dissection is close to the hepatic flexure, care must be exercised not to injure the gallbladder, or the duodenum. The best way to avoid injury is clear visualization of the duodenum and the gallbladder during dissection.

- Continue with the dissection until the hepatic flexure is completely down.

- Once this is complete, the right colon can be medialized up to the midline. The entire C-loop of the duodenum can be seen once the right colon is completely mobilized.

Mobilizing the Remaining Transverse Colon and Division of the Remaining Mesentery of the Transverse Colon

- At this point, the entire colon should be free for extraction except the transverse mesocolon.
- Place the patient in the reverse Trendelenburg position with the right side up. The surgeon should be on the patient's left side. Using the LLQ, and LUQ ports, continue with dividing the mesentery of the transverse colon. Continue with the division until the hepatic flexure. Middle colic vessels are ligated using the vessel-sealing device.
- Another option is to take the remaining mesentery of the transverse colon extracorporeally, which will save time; however, the incision should be adequate to control the mesentery. This is particularly useful in patients with a low BMI.

Exteriorization of the Specimen

- Prior to exteriorization, assess the mobility of the left, transverse, and right colon. All parts of the colon should now be in anatomical position to facilitate the exteriorization and prevent any twist while exteriorizing. One method of doing this is to grab the end of the specimen with a locking grasper and place another instrument under the colon and pull the entire colon over the second instrument making sure there are no attachments remaining.
- Use a locking grasper on the staple line of the distal sigmoid colon. Make sure that the bite is adequate, otherwise, when the locking grasper is moved toward the abdominal wall to exteriorize it, it might fall back into the abdomen, and then you have to re-insufflate the abdomen and search for it again. After the sigmoid colon is grasped, stop the insufflation.
- Extraction of the specimen.
  - Extraction from the midline: Remove the supraumbilical port. Extend the incision cranially and caudally. Limit the incision as much as possible. Remember, the incision can be extended as needed. Place a medium-sized wound protector.
    Alternatively:
  - Exteriorize from the proposed ileostomy site: This can be performed in patients who do not have a bulky specimen and who have a low-to-normal BMI. In addition, this would be suitable when all the mesenteric attachments are divided intracorporeally and there is nothing left apart from exteriorizing the specimen. The ileostomy site is fashioned as per routine and a medium wound protector is placed to facilitate extraction.
- Guide the laparoscopic locking grasper toward the extraction incision. Use a long Babcock forceps to grasp the staple line to exteriorize the specimen. Once that is done, release the laparoscopic locking grasper and pull it safely making sure that when you close the jaw of the laparoscopic grasper, it's under direct vision to avoid injury to any unintended structure (e.g., small bowel) that can get caught in the jaw of the grasper. Now, the specimen can be extracted gently.

Division of the Terminal Ileum and Creation of Stoma and Closure

- The terminal ileum (TI) is divided as close to the colon as possible using a blue load GIA stapler (3.8 mm).
- The 12-mm trocar in the RLQ should be removed, and the fascia should be incised as a cruciate incision, to accommodate two fingers.
- The surgeon now should pass the TI toward the RLQ. The assistant can use a Babcock forceps to grab the staple line of the TI and deliver it through the stoma site.

- Make sure the orientation is correct. This can be done by inserting an index finger through the abdominal wall just beside the stoma and feeling for the mesentery to make sure there are no twists. In addition, use the midline incision to inspect if there is any twist in the mesentery. Run the bowel to make sure of the orientation.

- Close the midline incision.

- The stoma should be matured in the usual standard fashion after the midline incision is closed.

- If the ileostomy site is used for extraction then the TI is divided, and the specimen passed off. Removal of the wound protector can sometimes be difficult. One can hold the end of the divided ileum with a Babcock forceps and lower it back into the wound while removing the wound protector. Alternatively, one can place a figure of eight stitch at the cut edge of the ileum and drop it back in the abdomen while holding the end of the stitch with a hemostat. Once the wound protector is out, the ileum can again be brought out and matured in the standard fashion. It is important to reconfirm the orientation and that there is no twist in the mesentery just before maturing the stoma. As a rule, we keep one 5-mm laparoscopic port in situ until the end of the surgery and if there is any doubt, we use a 5-mm camera to inspect the abdomen at the end of the operation.

Abdominal Operations

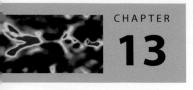

Laparoscopic Proctectomy and Creation of Ileal Pouch Anal Anastomosis

Ileal pouch anal anastomosis (IPAA) is the procedure of choice for restorative proctocolectomy. It is most commonly performed in cases of ulcerative colitis (UC) or familial adenomatous polyposis (FAP). In UC, the operation is often done in three stages, where the first operation will be the total abdominal colectomy with end ileostomy in patients who have severe disease, are malnourished, or are on a high dose of steroids or biologics. The second stage is done four to six months after the first operation. This allows the patient to recover from the first operation, regain their nutritional status, and stop the biologics and steroids. The second stage includes proctectomy, with the creation of the IPAA, and creation of the diverting loop ileostomy. The third stage is closure of the loop ileostomy. In this chapter, we describe the second stage of a three-stage pouch surgery, performed laparoscopically.

Preoperative Considerations

Ureteral Stents

In most cases, placement of ureteral stents is not necessary because the rectal inflammation tends to subside after the fecal diversion performed in the first stage. If severe scarring or inflammation is expected, then one must consider bilateral ureteral stents placement. It is particularly useful in patients who may have experienced rectal stump blow-out after their first stage and may have severe pelvic scarring.

Preoperative Steroids/Biologics

Steroids are commonly given in an acute flare. However, most patients are not on steroids or biologics during the second-stage surgery and so won't need stress dosing.

Stoma Marking

All these patients have an end ileostomy. The same site can be used for the loop ileostomy. In rare circumstances, the patient may have difficulty with their current ostomy. In these patients, one should have the ostomy nurse mark an ideal location for siting of the loop ileostomy. If necessary, this can be on the left side of the abdomen. It is usually not a problem to bring up the loop ileostomy on either side of the abdomen in these patients.

Obesity

It is very important to counsel the patient after their first-stage surgery to avoid gaining weight beyond their ideal body weight. Most of these patients regain their appetite and ability to absorb nutrients after their total colectomy and can easily gain excess weight beyond their presurgery weight or their ideal body weight. Another contributing factor is the advice to eat a low-fiber diet. It is important to explain to the patients that they can eat a regular diet a few weeks after their surgery and to give them a target weight. Patients who are obese will be at a higher risk for postoperative complications and have a higher likelihood of the pouch not reaching the top of the sphincters due to a thicker fat laden mesentery and a narrower pelvis. It is best to have them lose weight before doing the second-stage surgery.

Port Sites

- These patients have an end ileostomy in their right lower quadrant (RLQ). There are two ways to approach the surgery. One way is to take down the end ileostomy at the mucocutaneous junction taking care not to increase the skin opening as this site will be reused for the loop ileostomy. This approach is used when the surgeon does not anticipate any hindrance in completing the surgery (i.e., a "straightforward" case). Another approach is to start the surgery via a supraumbilical cut-down and use the four-port diamond-shaped configuration (Figure 13-1) to do the proctectomy first. This approach is used when a difficult proctectomy is anticipated (e.g., in patients who may have experienced rectal stump blow-out after their first stage and may have severe pelvic scarring) or in patients who have had multiple prior pelvic surgeries (e.g., those with endometriosis or prior prostate surgery). In this approach, once the surgeon is confident that the surgery can be completed, they can take down the ileostomy and use that site for extraction and pouch creation, if feasible.

- A periumbilical port (12 mm) is used for the camera.

- The RLQ and the suprapubic ports will be used to mobilize the rectum. Any energy source or laparoscopic scissors can be used to mobilize the rectum through the suprapubic port, while using an atraumatic grasper through the RLQ port to retract and provide better exposure.

- LLQ port: The initial dissection can be started with the above three ports. However, this port can be accessed by the second assistant who is standing across the surgeon, on the patient left side. The second assistant can use an atraumatic grasper to help retract the rectum out of the pelvis or provide countertraction during the dissection.

Abdominal Operations

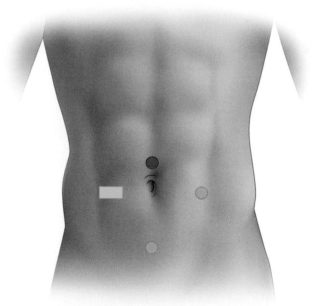

Figure 13-1. Port configuration in the proctectomy with creation of the IPAA. The green rectangle represents the old stoma site, the red circle represents the 12-mm camera, and the orange circles represent the 5-mm trocar sites.

Steps of the Operation

The steps of the operation are as follows:

- Ileostomy takedown.
- Creation of the ileal pouch.
- Lysis of adhesions.
- Proctectomy.
- Creation of the IPAA.
- Creation of a diverting loop ileostomy.

Ileostomy Takedown

- Start by closing the lumen of the small bowel. Take adequate bites to close it in a figure of eight fashion.
- Make a circular incision around the stoma at the mucocutaneous junction.
- After the stoma is taken down, and the adhesions are freed completely, extract the ileum to at least 40 cm. Choose a site of division as close to the stoma spout as possible. Divide the mesentery just next to this site.
- Divide the bowel at the chosen site just underneath the stoma spout to save as much small bowel as possible using a GIA stapler (we use a 3.5-mm thickness staple load).

Creation of the Ileal Pouch

- Fold the small bowel to create the J- pouch, where each limb is 15 cm.
- Align the two limbs by Placing three Lambert sutures, using 3-0 silk. A stitch should be placed between the tip of the blind end and the afferent limb. This will prevent elongation and folding of the blind loop with time.
- Longitudinal enterotomy is made at the apex of the J- pouch in the antimesenteric side.
- Place each limb of the GIA 100 stapler (3.5-mm thickness load, 100 mm in length) gently inside the bowel. Make sure that the mesentery is not involved in the staple line by checking posterior to the stapler, and making sure the mesentery on both limbs of bowel are directing away and not involved in the staple line.
- Fire the GIA stapler. After that, remove the "thicker" part of the stapler to get a new load, while keeping the "thinner" part inside. After that, push the thinner part further inside, and place the thicker part to the same level after it is advanced appropriately, and fire the stapler again.
- Typically, two fires suffice. Open the stapler and remove it gently.
- Check the staple line for any bleeding. A sponge stick without a sponge can be used to open the lumen of the bowel gently to visualize the whole staple line.
- Place a purse string stitch at the site of the enterotomy using 2-0 Prolene in the standard fashion.
- Place the anvil of the circular stapler inside the lumen of the pouch and tie the Prolene suture around securely. We use the 28-mm EEA stapler.
- Lambert sutures can be used to bury the staple line of the blind end of the J- pouch.
- Bring the apex of the pouch toward the symphysis pubis. If it reaches beyond the symphysis pubis, it indicates that the pouch should reach without tension during the anastomosis.

- Return the bowel to the abdominal cavity. This is sometimes tricky as the pouch is bulky for the ileostomy opening site and so one has to be very careful. Sometimes, it helps to place a small wound protector in order to "dilate" the abdominal wall and minimize friction while returning the pouch back into the abdominal cavity. Using warm, moist lap pads or warm saline also helps. At this stage of the surgery the patient needs to be completely relaxed. If, despite the above maneuvers, it is difficult to return the pouch safely into the abdomen, then one may have to increase the size of the fascial incision or skin opening. In this situation, it helps to place small (1–2 mm) release incisions at each quadrant of the circular skin incision instead of increasing its size circumferentially. This minimizes the problem of having a large diameter hole when maturing the loop ileostomy.

Lysis of Adhesions

- Close the fascial defect of the stoma site by using a PDS suture, in a figure of eight fashion, and prior to tying the sutures, place the Hasson trocar in between, and then tie. Alternatively, use a wound protector and place it inside the abdomen, and twist it around the Hasson trocar, and secure it with a 0-silk suture. Another alternative is to use a single incision port at this site.

- Place the other trocars under direct vision: a 12-mm (or 5-mm) port for the camera in the supraumbilical area, a 5-mm port in the suprapubic area, and a 5-mm port in the LLQ.

- We prefer using the 5-mm camera initially as it can be moved around from one port to the other when adhesions need to be lysed. In some patients with favorable anatomy, the operation can be completed using a single incision port at the ileostomy takedown site and a 5-mm supraumbilical camera port.

- In some patients it may be difficult to get visualization, but the surgeon may be able to perform some blunt finger dissection and feel the supraumbilical location by placing two fingers via the ileostomy takedown site. In this scenario, one can carefully place a 5-mm port right on their finger. This should only be done when the surgeon is sure that there are no structures adhered at that location and they can safely place the port "on their finger." It is important to place the port right on the surgeon's finger and not in between two fingers as it may impale the intestine if it slips in between the surgeon's fingers. The advantage of doing this when proper visualization from the ileostomy take down site is difficult is that one can place the 5-mm camera at this location and can get a different point of view, which can help with lysis of adhesions.

- Lysis of adhesions is done sharply to clear the abdominal wall, and pelvis. Laparoscopic peanuts may be used to do some gentle blunt dissection by an experienced surgeon. Sometimes, 5-mm ports may have to be placed at nonconventional locations in order to complete lysis of adhesions.

- Put the patient in the Trendelenburg position with the right side down.

- Reflect the small bowel out of the pelvis.

Proctectomy

- The rectal stump should be easily identified.

- In females, if the uterus is in the way, place a Keith needle beside the suprapubic port, and push it inside the abdominal cavity under laparoscopic guidance. Then take a bite in the uterus, and then out of the abdomen just beside the entry site of the needle. Tie the suture over a gauze piece. This will suspend the uterus up and away from the field of dissection (Figure 13-2).

- Start the rectal dissection by using laparoscopic scissors along the left pararectal sulcus. Use the RLQ port to provide appropriate traction, by holding the staple line of the rectal stump and pull it to the right side, while the second assistant on the left side of the bed can provide countertraction by an atraumatic grasper (Figure 13-3).

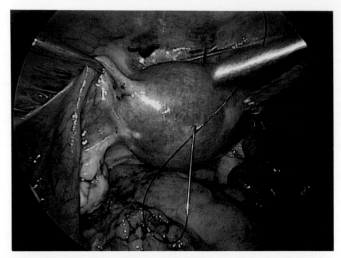

Figure 13-2. Suspending the uterus using a Keith needle that is inserted just beside the suprapubic port.

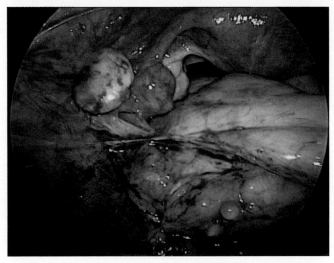

Figure 13-3. Retracting the rectal stump medially to start the dissection on the left pararectal sulcus.

- After scoring the peritoneum along the left pararectal sulcus, continue with the dissection deeper in the correct plane, being careful to identify and protect the ureter (Figures 13-4 to 13-6).

- Join the plane of dissection along the TME plane posteriorly. This plane should be bloodless (Figures 13-7 to 13-9).

- The advantage of dissecting along the TME plane is reduced blood loss and reduced risk of rectal injury. It is also ideal to remove the entire mesorectum if there is known or occult rectal cancer. However, it does increase the risk of injury to the pelvic autonomic nerves.

- The dissection should continue on the right pararectal sulcus in a similar fashion (Figure 13-10).

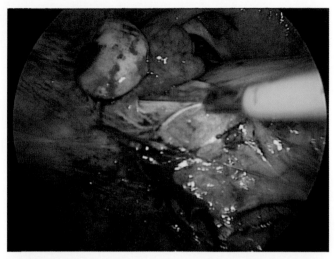

Figure 13-4. Starting the dissection along the left pararectal sulcus. Extreme care should be exercised to avoid injuring the left ureter.

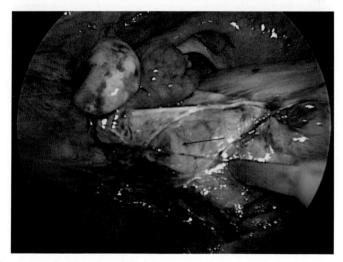

Figure 13-5. The arrow is showing where the left ureter is, which is very close to the line of the dissection.

- Finally, the anterior plane should be dissected. In females, consider placing a vaginal probe and lift it up to facilitate the identification of the vagina. Use the laparoscopic scissors and score the plane anteriorly, and push the vagina upward and away from the rectum.
- The dissection should be continued until the pelvic floor is reached (Figure 13-11).
- An Endo GIA stapler is used through the RLQ port to divide the rectum, preferable in one firing. We use the 60-mm length 3.5-mm thickness Endo GIA stapler (Figure 13-12).
- If there are any remaining mesenteric attachments, it can be taken down using LigaSure.
- The rectum should now be completely dissected. Remove it from the pelvis, and place it in the RLQ.

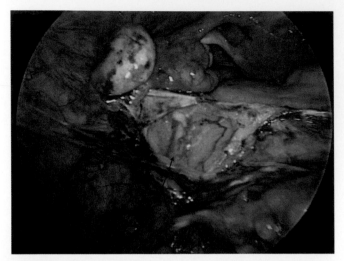

Figure 13-6. Further dissection showed the course of the left ureter. Note that this is not the correct plane of dissection that should be more medial to this plane.

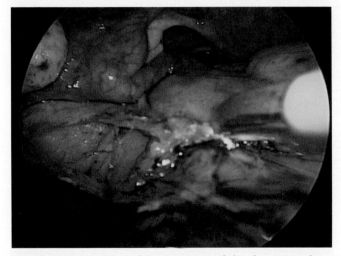

Figure 13-7. Restoring the appropriate plane of dissection just medial to the previous dissection plane.

Creation of the Anastomosis

- Bring the pouch down toward the pelvis.
- If there is any tension in the pouch to bring it down, consider the following:
  - ○ Complete adhesiolysis.
  - ○ Make sure the mesentery of the small bowel is mobilized up to the duodenojejunal junction.
  - ○ Score the peritoneum over the superior mesenteric artery (SMA) anteriorly and posteriorly.
  - ○ Division of the terminal branches of the SMA or ileocolic artery given that the blood supply to the terminal ileum is not compromised. Clamping of the vessel for 15 minutes is recommended prior to the division of the vessel.
  - ○ Consider using an S-pouch instead of a J-pouch.

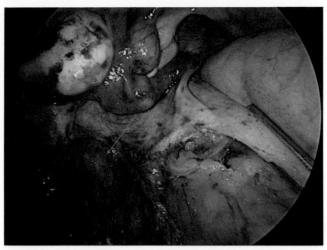

Figure 13-8. The orange arrow showing the old wrong plane, and the blue arrow showing the correct dissection plane.

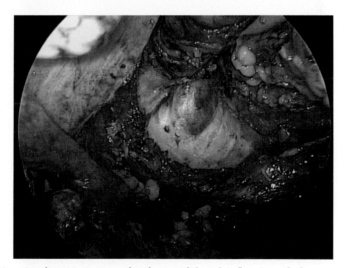

Figure 13-9. Dissecting the posterior avascular plane until the pelvic floor is reached.

- Place the EEA circular stapler size 28 in the anal canal very carefully. It is important to gently dilate the sphincters to two fingers and use blunt sizers to dilate the sphincters to the appropriate size and then introduce the stapler in a fully controlled fashion to avoid disrupting the short anorectal stump. This should be performed by an experienced surgeon/senior surgical trainee.
- Prior to firing the stapler, make sure of the following points:
  - No twist in the mesentery. Ideally, the pouch is anterior with the mesentery posterior. Sometimes this is not possible anatomically and the mesentery may sit on one side. Although not ideal, it is acceptable.
  - If no tension, join the anvil with the spike.

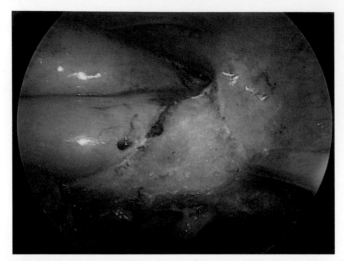

Figure 13-10. Pulling the rectum to the left side, while scoring the anterior plane to join the already dissected anterior plane from the left side.

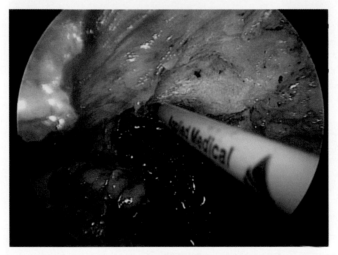

Figure 13-11. Continuing with the dissection circumferentially until the pelvis floor is reached.

○ Close the stapler, making sure the vagina is completely out of the way. Vaginal exam can be helpful to make sure that it's away from the stapler. After the stapler is closed, the vaginal exam should be repeated, and with gentle movement of the stapler. If the vagina is caught in the stapler, there will be a sensation of movement or puckering of the vagina. If this happens, then the stapler should be opened, the vagina retracted anteriorly while the stapler is closed again, and check again to make sure the vagina is not pinched. At this point if there is any doubt then further mobilization of the vagina may need to be carried out.

• Once the stapler is closed and the vagina is clear, fire the stapler. We wait 20 seconds before removing the stapler. One must follow the guidelines from the individual stapler manufacturers with regards to firing and removal.

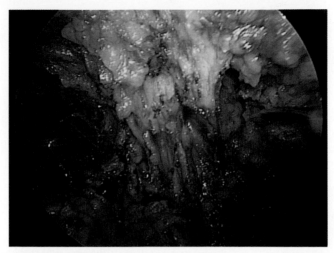

Figure 13-12. Preparing for stapling at the level of the pelvic floor.

Creation of a Diverting Loop Ileostomy

- The patient is repositioned to right side up.

- Follow the small bowel from the pouch proximally, to choose a loop of small bowel that can be brought up for creation of diverting loop ileostomy, usually 20–30 cm from the pouch.

- Make sure that the loop is reaching the abdominal wall without any tension, and the orientation is correct.

- A locking grasper is used to hold the stapler line in the rectum. Another bowel grasper is used to hold the medial edge of the mesentery of the chosen loop of small bowel to be brought out as an ileostomy.

- Desufflate the abdomen.

- Use the stoma site to remove the rectum, and then bring the loop of small bowel up for stoma creation.

- A bowel clamp can be placed on the exteriorized small bowel to hold it in place, and prevent any twist.

- Reestablish pneumoperitoneum again.

- Make sure the orientation of the bowel is correct. Check for hemostasis.

- Remove the suture that was holding the uterus. Make sure the site of the needle entry in the uterus is not bleeding. This will require to lift up the uterus using atraumatic grasper to make sure there is no bleeding. Monopolar scissors may be used to achieve hemostasis.

- Remove all trocars under direct supervision.

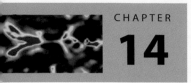

14 Laparoscopic Rectopexy

Laparoscopic rectopexy, with or without resection of the sigmoid colon, is one of the surgical options to treat rectal prolapse. In addition to the rectopexy, a sigmoid resection is recommended in patients who have constipation preoperatively, as the rectopexy alone may worsen the constipation symptoms.

Preoperative Considerations

Ureteral Stents

Usually, straightforward laparoscopic rectopexy does not need ureteral stent placement. However, in some cases with large, chronic rectal prolapse, the ureter might be more medial than expected due to traction and tissue laxity predisposing to ureteral injury.

Port Sites

Four Port Diamond-Shaped Configuration (Figure 14-1)

- This configuration will allow you to do any colon or rectal operation.
- A periumbilical port (12 mm) is used for the camera.
- The right lower quadrant (RLQ) and the suprapubic ports will be used to mobilize the rectum. An energy source or laparoscopic scissors with monopolar cautery can be used to mobilize the rectum through the suprapubic port, while using an atraumatic grasper through the RLQ port to retract and provide better exposure.
- Left lower quadrant (LLQ) port: The initial dissection can be started with the above three ports. However, a second assistant who is standing in front of the surgeon, on the patient's left side, can use this port. The second assistant can use an atraumatic grasper to help with retracting the rectum out of the pelvis or provide countertraction during the dissection.

Steps of the Operation

- General steps.
- Exposure of the pelvis.
- Rectal dissection.
- Resection rectopexy.
- Fixation of the rectum.

Exposure of the Pelvis

Adhesiolysis may be needed in patients who have had prior surgery. The uterus may need to be suspended for proper exposure (Figures 14-2 and 14-3).

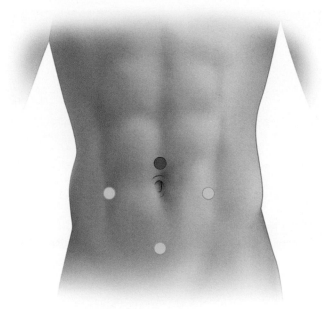

Figure 14-1. Four ports diamond-shaped configuration. Supraumbilical 12-mm site for the camera, and the rest are 5-mm ports.

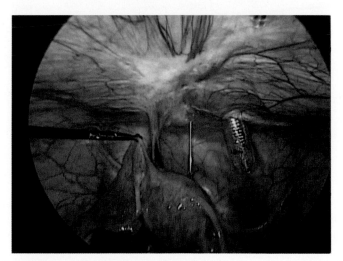

Figure 14-2. Before starting with the pelvic dissection, the uterus is suspended to the abdominal wall by inserting a Keith needle just beside the suprapubic port to suspend the uterus.

Rectal Dissection (Figures 14-4 to 14-15)

- Place the patient in the steep Trendelenburg position with the right side down.
- Reflect the omentum over the transverse colon.

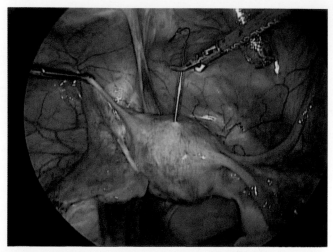

Figure 14-3. The needle is inserted through the body of the uterus and then the needle is directed toward the abdominal wall again.

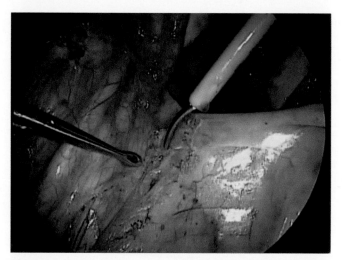

Figure 14-4. Starting the rectal dissection by retracting the rectum out of the pelvis and toward the right side, to dissect the left pararectal sulcus.

- Start the rectal dissection by scoring the peritoneum in the left pararectal sulcus from the level of the sacral promontory downward. The dissection can be done using laparoscopic scissors with monopolar cautery through the suprapubic port, while using an atraumatic grasper to retract the rectum medially. The second assistant can provide counter traction by placing an atraumatic grasper through the LLQ port and hold the peritoneum in the left pelvic wall and pull it laterally. The left ureter should be identified and protected at all the time. Be mindful that the location of both ureters could be more medial due to the chronic prolapse.

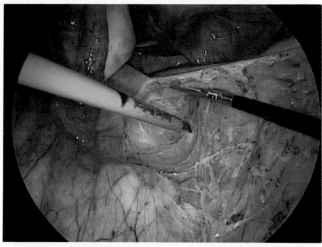

Figure 14-5. Starting the posterior dissection from the left side of the rectum after the TME plane is entered.

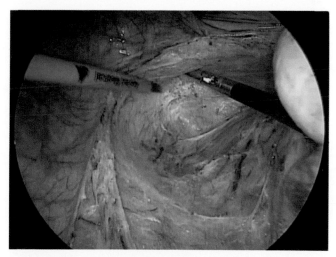

Figure 14-6. Continuing the dissection toward the pelvic floor through the TME (avascular) plane.

- After the left pararectal sulcus is scored, the dissection is continued deeper, until the presacral space is entered from the left side. During low anterior resection, the presacral space is entered easily after the medial dissection is done, and the IMA is divided. However, during rectopexy, the IMA is preserved and the medial dissection is not needed.

- The right pararectal sulcus is scored in a similar fashion. The surgeon uses the energy source through the suprapubic port, while the second assistant retracts the rectum to the left side. The presacral plane is entered from the right side and the dissection planes are joined.

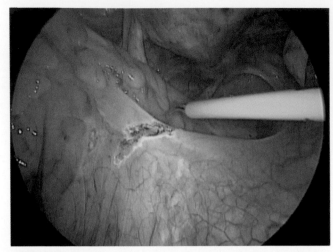

Figure 14-7. Starting scoring the sigmoid colon medially toward the pelvis in the avascular plane.

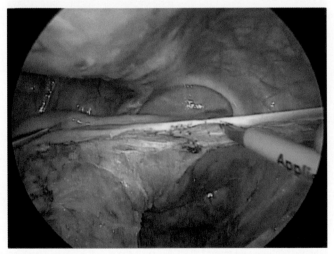

Figure 14-8. Scoring the right pararectal sulcus using laparoscopic scissors, while retracting the rectum out of the pelvis and toward the left.

- The dissection posteriorly should be continued in the total mesorectal excision (TME) plane until the pelvic floor is reached. The hypogastric nerves should be preserved to avoid any sexual or bladder dysfunction.
- The lateral rectal stalks should be preserved because their division may lead to denervation of the rectum that leads to constipation. However, this theory has been challenged. Therefore, if the whole rectum can be pulled up and the prolapse is completely reduced without division of the lateral stalks, then it's best to avoid it.

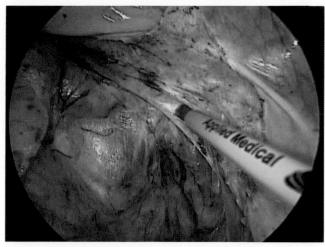

Figure 14-9. The dissection is continued down toward the pelvis while retracting the pelvis up and out of the pelvis.

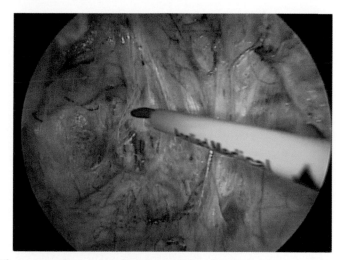

Figure 14-10. The posterior dissection is continued until the pelvic floor as demonstrated is reached.

- The anterior plane is scored at the level of the peritoneal reflection. This step is difficult due to a deep cul-de-sac. In females, and due to chronic rectal prolapse, the vaginal wall is sometimes abnormally fused to the rectum leading to more difficult dissection. The anterior dissection should be continued until the dissection reaches the pelvic floor circumferentially.

- Perform a digital rectal examination, which will confirm that the rectal dissection is low enough at the pelvic floor.

- In females, consider doing a vaginal exam as well to make sure that the vaginal cuff is dissected away from the rectum.

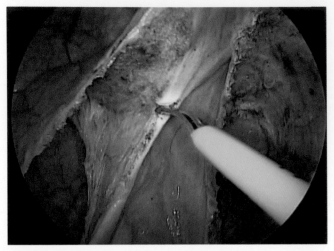

Figure 14-11. Dissecting the anterior plane using laparoscopic scissors and dissecting the vagina away from the anterior plane from the rectum.

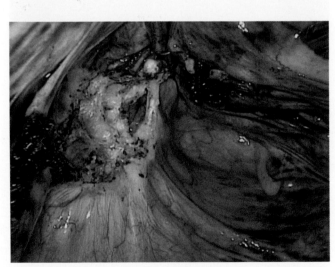

Figure 14-12. In a different case, due to extensive fibrosis between the vagina and the anterior wall of the rectum, there was a vaginal injury.

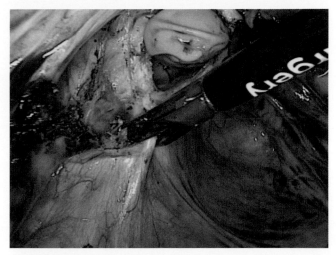

Figure 14-13. Using the defect in the vagina, an index finger is placed in the vagina, to retract it upward to help delineate the plane between the vagina and the anterior wall of the rectum.

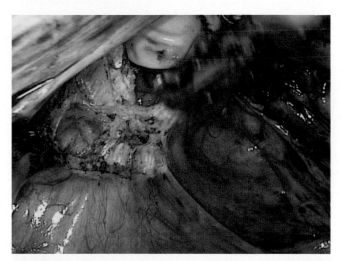

Figure 14-14. The dissection in the anterior dissection is continued. Notice the amount of fibrosis in that plane due to chronic prolapse.

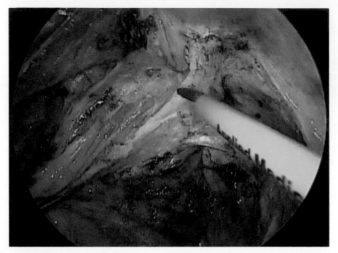

Figure 14-15. Dissecting the anterior plane circumferentially until the pelvic floor is reached.

Resection Rectopexy (Figures 14-16 to 14-18)

- The sigmoid resection is performed as described in the sigmoid resection chapter.
- The key is to perform the rectopexy stitches after the anastomosis is made.
- During the rectopexy stitch placement, only the top of the rectum should be handled. The colon leading up to the colorectal anastomosis should not be pulled or retracted because it could disrupt the anastomosis.
- The leak test should be performed twice—once after the anastomosis is made and once after the rectopexy is completed.

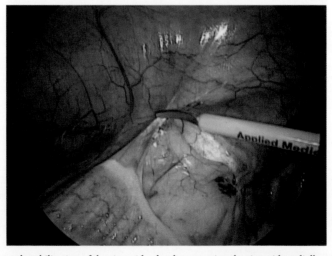

Figure 14-16. Lateral mobilization of the sigmoid colon by retracting the sigmoid medially using the RLQ port, and dividing the attachments through the suprapubic port.

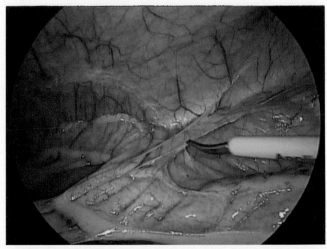

Figure 14-17. Further mobilization of the sigmoid colon toward the splenic flexure. Further mobilization would be required if resection of the sigmoid colon will be performed with the rectopexy.

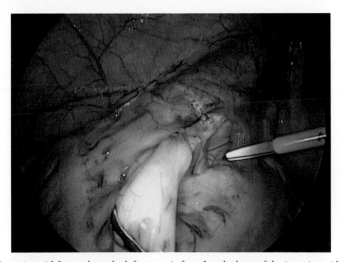

Figure 14-18. Intersigmoid fossa where the left ureter is found at the base of the intersigmoid fossa.

Fixation of the Rectum

- After the rectum is dissected, the rectum should be pulled out of the pelvis, to reduce the prolapse and it should be straight without any redundancy.
- Using the lateral rectal stalks, the rectum should be fixed to sacral promontory, 1 cm off midline to avoid injury to the sacral vessels that are in the midline (Figures 14-19 and 14-20).
- Fixation can be done using a ProTack Fixation Device or suturing using nonabsorbable sutures. Alternatively, an extracorporeal Roeder's knot can be used and pushed using a knot pusher. A Roeder's knot is a sliding knot, which consists of one hitch, three winds, and one locking hitch (1:3:1) (Figure 14-21).

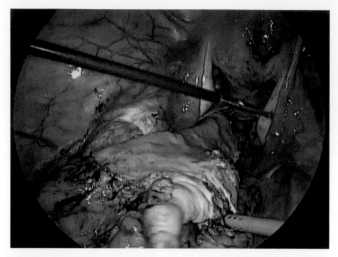

Figure 14-19. After sigmoid resection and handsewn colorectal anastomosis, the rectum below the anastomosis is lifted up to the level of the sacral promontory in order to fix it to the sacral promontory.

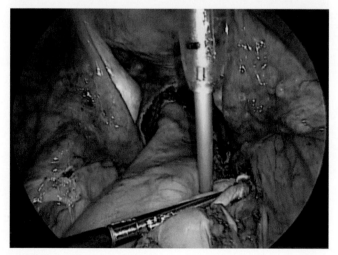

Figure 14-20. After sigmoid resection and handsewn colorectal anastomosis, the rectum below the anastomosis is lifted up to the level of the sacral promontory and a laparoscopic tacker is used to fix it just off the midline.

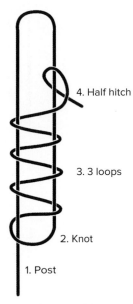

4. Half hitch

3. 3 loops

2. Knot

1. Post

Figure 14-21. Diagrammatic representation of the Roeder's knot.

Dealing with Complications and Difficulties in Colon and Rectal Surgery

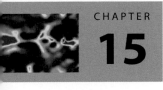

CHAPTER

15 Presacral Bleeding

One of the rare, yet major complications that can occur during rectal dissection is presacral bleeding. This injury can result in massive blood loss, hemodynamic instability, and even death.

An anatomical study was carried out across 100 pieces of sacrum to study the anatomy of the presacral venous plexus. They found that in 16% of the specimens, there were one to several large foramina, which are the sites for the basivertebral veins to penetrate. In other specimens, these foramina were very small. These are located at the level of S3–S5.[1] The adventitia of these presacral veins is attached to the sacral periosteum at the openings of these foramina. This explains why these veins can be injured during blunt dissection of the rectum, where the surgeon retracts the rectum anteriorly and bluntly dissects through the posterior plane, and will pull on the presacral fascia and injure these delicate veins near their foramina. These veins, consequently, will retract inside the bone, and will cause massive bleeding.

The presacral venous plexus is located anterior to the sacrum, and it is formed by two lateral presacral veins, and the middle sacral vein. These are interconnected by communicating veins. The presacral venous plexus is connected to the internal vertebral venous system through the basivertebral veins that pass through the sacral foramina.

Patterns of Injury

Wang et al.[1] classified the patterns of presacral vein injury to three different types: (1) bleeding from injury to the presacral venous plexus, (2) bleeding from the pelvic surface of the distal sacrum, and (3) bleeding from an injury to a large caliber sacral basivertebral vein (Figure 15-1).

The amount of bleeding depends on the size of the vessel injured, and the hydrostatic pressure in the sacral venous plexus. The lithotomy position can increase the hydrostatic pressure up to double or triple the pressure in the inferior vena cava, and thus lead to more profuse bleeding.[1] In addition, due to the lack of valves in this complex venous network, this will make the bleeding even worse.

Risk Factors and Mechanism of Injury

Risk factors that might lead to this injury could be related to anatomical factors or technical factors. Anatomical factors are those such as a very narrow pelvis or severe fibrosis in the dissection planes posteriorly secondary to the radiation effects leading to fixation of the posterior rectum to the anterior surface of the sacrum.[2] Additional risk factors include recurrent rectal cancer, or extension of the tumor posteriorly. There are few intraoperative technical errors that lead to this injury.

1. The surgeon may be in the wrong plane where the dissection is too posterior.

2. Blunt dissection in the posterior plane, which is considered one of the common mechanisms of such an injury. This is because the adventitia of these veins are attached to the sacral periosteum, and blunt dissection will rip off the vein(s) causing massive bleeding.[1]

3. Attempting to hold the vessels in the presacral fascia and lifting it or trying to suture it in the usual fashion will aggravate the bleeding, because these veins are delicate and can tear very easily and consequently retract in the sacral foramina and cause massive bleeding.[1]

4. Being in the wrong plane too posterior from the perineal part, while doing an abdominoperineal will cause this injury as well.

Injury to the presacral veins will cause massive bleeding that is difficult to control using usual hemostatic techniques. This complication can be even more difficult to manage when this is encountered robotically or laparoscopically. When this complication happens, there are a few steps that should be carried out immediately. Conversion to lower midline laparotomy is done in a timely fashion, unless the bleeding can be controlled quickly and safely using minimally invasive techniques.

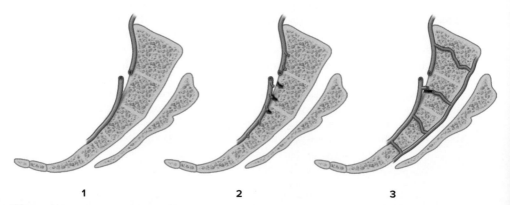

Figure 15-1. Three types of presacral vein injury.

Management of Presacral Bleeding

There are different reported methods and techniques to control presacral bleeding. However, the initial goals to manage this problem are the same.

1. Apply direct pressure to the bleeding area to stop or slow down the rate of bleeding. This can be achieved using laparotomy pads, direct pressure with finger(s), a small tampon gauze, or an absorbable knitted fabric hemostat.[2]

2. Decrease the lithotomy position by lowering the legs especially if the legs were positioned high, since this will decrease the pressure in the presacral venous plexus.

3. Both the anesthesia and nursing teams should be notified promptly about the situation. This will avoid dealing with a major catastrophe while the other members of the team are distracted with other less essential issues.

4. Ask for extra help. An extra nurse can be added to the team to help bring unusual or unexpected instruments that will be required to control the bleeding, especially if there was no designed kit for presacral bleeding. Asking for help also includes asking for the assistance of a senior surgeon if available, or another colleague to help if needed. Keep in mind that asking for help early is very critical.

5. If the hospital has a massive transfusion protocol, then that can be initiated in conjunction with the anesthesia team.

6. Ask for additional adjuncts such as extra suction units with its tubing to allow effective suctioning, and headlights. The extra suction device will allow very rapid evacuation of the blood in order to identify the bleeding site.

Now, the decision should be made to choose which is the definitive method to control this bleeding.

Packing

The first thing to be done is to quickly pack the pelvis with laparotomy pads and apply pressure. If the bleeding is controlled with direct pressure, continue holding, and proceed with the rectal dissection and get the specimen out. This will give the surgeon more space, especially in case where the pelvis is narrow.

If the patient is unstable, this can be managed as "damage control" where the pelvis is packed, and the abdomen is temporarily closed if the packing is controlling the bleeding. Send the patient for surgical intensive care unit for continued resuscitation, and bring the patient back to the operating room (OR) after 24 hours, for removal of the packing, and creation of the anastomosis.[3] The disadvantages of this technique are the requirement of reoperation to remove the pelvic packing, and then perform the anastomosis. In addition, it will be difficult to detect if the bleeding has started again. Risk of infection is low since the packing will be removed within 24 to 48 hours.

A modified packing technique has been described, where a small intestinal isolation bag is inserted in the pelvic cavity through the perineum. Rolled gauze is inserted in the bowel plastic bag. The perineal wound is closed around the bag with the neck of the bag and strings exposed.[4] This modification has few advantages. First the gauze will not absorb the blood if the patient started to bleed, but rather, the bleeding will come out of the perineal wound. In addition, removal of the packing can be at bedside, and it can be done gradually, by removing a couple of sponges first, and then removal of the remaining one, with the intestinal bag.[4] Another technique is to use a four lumen Sengstaken-Blakemore tube to control the bleeding.[5] The tube is placed from the perineal wound, and then the gastric balloon is inflated with air to a volume adequate for compression of the presacral region, and distal traction is applied.[5] Another technique that can be used is to place a saline bag through the perineal port. The saline bag has a port for infusion of the saline. This technique has few advantages.

The amount of pressure will be controlled by the amount of saline that is instilled in the bag. In addition, the saline bag can be removed at bedside. It's always available in the OR, and it's not costly.[6] Tissue expanders have been used as well, with similar results.[7]

Epiploica or Muscle Welding

An epiploica or omental tag can be used and applied directly to the bleeding point using a long DeBakey forceps, or a laparoscopic grasper. Then, electrocautery is applied to the metal part of the grasper to cauterize the epiploica. Using a piece of epiploica to control the bleeding has couple of advantages. Applying direct electrocautery to the bleeding area will not control the bleeding given that the blood will be a barrier in between the bleeding area or vessel and the tip of the electrocautery, which will not conduct appropriately. In addition, with the massive bleeding, visualization of the bleeding site will be very poor, and the operator will not know where to apply the electrocautery.

Muscle fragment welding has been described as well. A 2-cm square segment of the rectus muscle is harvested and held with a forceps over the site of bleeding. Adequate use of suction is mandatory to visualize the site of the bleeding. Electrocautery is used at a high setting (100 Hz) on the instrument. The effect will be welding the bleeding site with that muscle fragment.[8] Another technique using the rectus muscle is to control the bleeding with packing, and then place two sutures on each side of the bleeding point. Then, the muscle is placed on the top of the bleeding site, and the two sutures are tied.[9]

Thumbtacks

Sterile metallic or titanium thumbtacks have been used successfully to control massive presacral bleeding. By holding the thumbtack using a needle holder or a Kelly clamp, it's directly placed in the sacral foramina where the bleeding is coming from.[1,10,11] Prior to that, adequate suctioning should be ready when the pressure by finger or sponge is removed to help determine the exact location of the site of bleeding. The downside of this technique is the placement of a foreign body permanently in the patient, with unknown consequences of this technique in the long term. In addition, this technique will not be effective if the bleeding source is diffuse or coming from multiple sites. Moreover, placing the thumbtack very low in the pelvis, where the site of the bleeding usually is, is technically difficult especially in a narrow pelvis, with the natural pelvic curvature, which are all factors that make this technique difficult.

Bone Wax

Bone wax should be readily available in most ORs, and can be easily applied to the presacral area to decrease or stop the bleeding. The bone wax can be used alone, or in conjunction with other techniques such as packing to stop the bleeding completely.[12]

Circular Suture Ligation

Usually, direct suture ligation of the bleeding presacral veins is futile. However, this technique has been reported to be effective.[13] Suture ligation in circles around the bleeding site has been reported to be effective, using a 4-0 silk suture with a narrow-tapered needle. The suture bite should include the presacral fascia, the presacral veins, and the deep connective tissues. If this controlled the bleeding, Surgicel can be placed on top of the area. If the bleeding persists, then another circular suture ligation is performed inside the bigger circle.

Electrocautery

Conventional ways to control bleeding usually does not work with presacral bleeding. However, it was reported that using the spray mode of electrocautery, 3–5 mm away from the bleeding vessels at a 90° angle can be helpful to control the presacral bleeding.

Argon Beam Coagulation

Argon beam coagulation (ABC) is a monopolar electrosurgical technique that uses argon discharges at atmospheric pressure to coagulate tissue.[14] It has many advantages. It is quick and available in the OR. In addition, it can be used laparoscopically as well. Rapid coagulation is achieved because the flow of argon gas clears the target site of blood. This is an important feature in the ABC where the operator can locate the exact bleeding site, and target the beam toward that area. In addition, the even and consistent application of energy through the ionized argon beam seals the tissue.[15] Reported complications from the ABC is venous argon embolism.[16] To avoid such a complication, the probe should not be in direct contact with the tissue, and it should be a few millimeters away. In addition, limit argon flow settings to the lowest levels that will provide the desired clinical effect. Also, hold the tip of the electrode at an oblique angle; purge the gas line of air before each procedure; and move the hand piece away from the tissue after each activation.[16]

Infra-Renal Aortic Control

After the initial measures are taken, including placing pressure by fingers or sponges to the bleeding area, the peritoneum over the aorta is opened, and the aorta just above the bifurcation is clamped. This will decrease the arterial blood flow to the pelvis and lower extremities, which consequently will decrease the venous return and thus the bleeding. The decrease in the rate of the bleeding will allow the surgeon to identify the site of the bleeding exactly, and allowing the surgeon to apply any direct technique such as direct suturing, thumbtack, etc.[17] This must be done in conjunction with vascular surgery and the standard protocols used for clamping major vessels (use of heparin, etc.) must be followed.

Other Techniques

There are other reported techniques to control presacral bleeding.

One technique is to fold the Surgicel to 2.5 × 2.5 cm in size and place it directly over the bleeding point. The Surgicel is fixed into the sacrum using the ProTack.[18] Another technique is to use the expanded polytetrafluoroethylene (PTFE) pledgets to control the bleeding, and then fix to the sacrum using the ProTack.[19] Using the ProTack has a few advantages. It's widely available in most ORs. It is easy to use, and has many loads that can be used repetitively without moving the PTFE, or Surgicel. In addition, it can be used in open and laparoscopic cases. Finally, it will allow the operator to place the ProTacks even with difficult angles deep in the pelvis.

Another technique is to use a bone graft at the site of the bleeding together with Surgicel to control the bleeding, and fix into the sacrum using a table fixation staple.[20] This technique requires the presence of specialized orthopedic instruments in the OR: staple hammer, staple driver, table fixation staple, bone graft, and Surgicel.[20] The advantage of this technique that it can be used to tamponade the bleeding when the defect in the sacrum is too large for the thumbtack.

Another technique is to use a few pieces of Surgicel folded by a Kelly clamp, and placed directly to the bleeding site, followed by Cyanoacrylate glue to fix it to the bleeding site.[21] Another technique is to use hemostatic sponge and cyanoacrylate glue to control the bleeding.[22]

Other combinations of hemostatic agents have been used successfully. It was reported that a combination of hemostatic matrix (FloSeal; Baxter, USA) and an absorbable hemostat (Surgicel Fibrillar; Ethicon, USA) together is an effective method to control presacral bleeding. One of its advantages is that it's readily available in the OR, and easy to use.[23]

It was even reported that using the endoscopic stapling device (Endopath EMS, Endoscopic multifeed stapler, Ethicon, Inc.) can be used to directly place the titanium staples at the point of bleeding and these staples will compress the vein against the bone.[24]

Dealing with Complications and Difficulties in Colon and Rectal Surgery

Ligation of the Internal Iliac Artery or Vein

Ligation of the internal iliac artery could be thought as a logical step to decrease or control presacral bleeding. However, ligation of the internal iliac artery will not affect the hydrostatic pressure within the sacral venous system, resulting in persistent bleeding. Moreover, it was reported that it may lead to necrosis of the buttock and the urinary bladder.[25] Ligation of the internal iliac vein will worsen the bleeding even further, because of the resulting blockage of the venous drainage from the pelvic, gluteal, and obturator veins, and redirecting the blood through the lateral sacral veins toward the injured vein.[26]

Summary

In conclusion, presacral bleeding is a rare complication in rectal surgery. There is no single "best method" to control presacral bleeding, which makes it important for the surgeon to be aware of the various options. Having a plan in mind will be helpful during a major catastrophe in the OR. It's also a good idea to have ready some of the simple items that are usually not present in a colorectal OR, such as a sterilized thumbtack, or bone wax in a specialized box for emergencies.

REFERENCES

1. Wang QY, Shi WJ, Zhao YR, Zhou WQ, He ZR. New concepts in severe presacral hemorrhage during proctectomy. *Arch Surg.* 1985;120(9):1013-1020.

2. D'Ambra L, Berti S, Bonfante P, Bianchi C, Gianquinto D, Falco E. Hemostatic step-by-step procedure to control presacral bleeding during laparoscopic total mesorectal excision. *World J Surg.* 2009;33(4):812-815.

3. Tarquini VC, et al. Pelvic packing: a rescue treatment for severe presacral hemorrhage. *Eur Surg.* 2012;44(2):124-125.

4. Metzger PP, Modified packing technique for control of presacral pelvic bleeding. *Dis Colon Rectum.* 1988;31(12):981-982.

5. McCourtney JS, Hussain N, Mackenzie I. Balloon tamponade for control of massive presacral haemorrhage. *Br J Surg.* 1996;83(2):222.

6. Ng X, Chiou W, Chang S. Controlling a presacral hemorrhage by using a saline bag: report of a case. *Dis Colon Rectum.* 2008;51(6):972-974.

7. Cosman BC, Lackides GA, Fisher DP, Eskenazi LB. Use of tissue expander for tamponade of presacral hemorrhage. Report of a case. *Dis Colon Rectum.* 1994;37(7):723-726.

8. Harrison JL, Hooks VH, Pearl RK, et al. Muscle fragment welding for control of massive presacral bleeding during rectal mobilization: a review of eight cases. *Dis Colon Rectum.* 2003;46(8):1115-1117.

9. Remzi FH, Oncel M, Fazio VW. Muscle tamponade to control presacral venous bleeding: report of two cases. *Dis Colon Rectum.* 2002;45(8):1109-1111.

10. Nivatvongs S, Fang DT. The use of thumbtacks to stop massive presacral hemorrhage. *Dis Colon Rectum.* 1986;29(9):589-590.

11. Stewart BT, McLaughlin SJ. Control of pre-sacral haemorrhage by drawing pin tamponade. *Aust N Z J Surg.* 1996;66(10):715-716.

12. Civelek A, Yegen C, Aktan AO. The use of bone-wax to control massive presacral bleeding. *Surg Today.* 2002;32(10):944-945.

13. Jiang J, Li X, Wang Y, Qu H, Jin Z, Dai Y. Circular suture ligation of presacral venous plexus to control presacral venous bleeding during rectal mobilization. *J Gastrointest Surg.* 2013;17(2):416-420.

14. Zenker M. Argon plasma coagulation. *GMS Krankenhhyg Interdiszip.* 2008;3(1):Doc15.

15. Saurabh S, Strobos EH, Patankar S, Zinkin L, Kassir A, Snyder M. The argon beam coagulator: a more effective and expeditious way to address presacral bleeding. *Tech Coloproctol.* 2014;18(1):73-76.

16. Stojeba N, Mahoudeau G, Segura P, Meyer C, Steib A. Possible venous argon gas embolism complicating argon gas enhanced coagulation during liver surgery. *Acta Anaesthesiol Scand.* 1999;43(8):866-867.

17. Papalambros E, Sigala F, Felekouras E, et al. Management of massive presacral bleeding during low pelvic surgery – an alternative technique. *Zentralbl Chir.* 2005;130(3):267-269.

18. Nasralla D, Lucarotti M. An innovative method for controlling presacral bleeding. *Ann R Coll Surg Engl.* 2013;95(5):375-376.

19. Joseph P, Perakath B. Control of presacral venous bleeding with helical tacks on PTFE pledgets combined with pelvic packing. *Tech Coloproctol.* 2011;15(1):79-80.

20. Wang LT, Feng CC, Wu CC, Hsiao CW, Weng PW, Jao SW. The use of table fixation staples to control massive presacral hemorrhage: a successful alternative treatment. Report of a case. *Dis Colon Rectum.* 2009;52(1):159-161.

21. Chen Y, Chen F, Xie P, Qiu P, Zhou J, Deng Y. Combined oxidized cellulose and cyanoacrylate glue in the management of severe presacral bleeding. *Surg Today.* 2009;39(11):1016-1017.

22. Losanoff JE, Richman BW, Jones JW. Cyanoacrylate adhesive in management of severe presacral bleeding. *Dis Colon Rectum.* 2002; 45(8):1118-1119.

23. Germanos S, Bolanis I, Saedon M, Baratsis S. Control of presacral venous bleeding during rectal surgery. *Am J Surg.* 2010;200(2):e33-35.

24. Celentano V, Ausobsky JR, Vowden P. Surgical management of presacral bleeding. *Ann R Coll Surg Engl.* 2014;96(4):261-265.

25. Tajes RV. Ligation of the hypogastric arteries and its complication in resection of cancer of the rectum. *Am J Gastroenterol.* 1956;26(5):612-618.

26. Filippakis GM, Leandros M, Albanopoulos K, et al. The use of spray electrocautery to control presacral bleeding: a report of four cases. *Am Surg.* 2007;73(4):410-413.

Dealing with Complications and Difficulties in Colon and Rectal Surgery

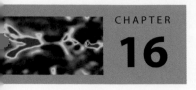

Difficulties with Reach During Construction of Colorectal Anastomosis

One of the basic principles of creating a healthy anastomosis is to make sure it is tension free. In most cases, this can be achieved. However, in certain conditions, creating a tension-free anastomosis is difficult and may not be possible. There are a few risk factors that could lead to this problem, including prior history of colectomy, extensive resection of the left colon, inadequate blood supply of the left colon, and lack of redundancy of the colon, or a short colon.

In these cases, the standard technique for mobilization may not be enough to achieve a tension-free colorectal anastomosis.

Make sure the following steps have been completed:

- The splenic flexure should be completely mobilized. This can be achieved by mobilizing the splenic flexure in antegrade and retrograde fashion.

- Division of the inferior mesenteric artery (IMA) at its origin close to the aorta will allow for more reach of the left colon to ensure tension-free anastomosis. However, attention should be paid to make sure that the colon that will be brought to the pelvis for the anastomosis has adequate blood supply.

- The next step after IMA division is division of the inferior mesenteric vein (IMV) at the inferior border of the pancreas.

- Mobilize the transverse colon, and divide the omentum off the transverse colon.

After completion of the above maneuvers, if there is inadequate length of the proximal colon to bring down to make an anastomosis to the rectum then one has the following options:

1. Consider mobilizing the rectum in the total mesorectal excision (TME) plane. This can provide a few centimeters of length without compromising the blood supply of the rectum.

2. Consider dividing the middle colic vessels if they are the limiting factor. After complete mobilization of the splenic flexure with division of the IMV, IMA, and rectal mobilization, typically the point of "tension" is at the middle colic vessels. They will need to be divided at this time to get adequate length.

3. After division of the middle colic vessels, there are two ways to bring the colon down into the pelvis in order to make the anastomosis. One is to bring the colon through the small intestine mesentery and the other is to completely mobilize the right colon and rotate it counterclockwise (Deloyer's procedure). The ideal approach will depend on how much colon has been resected, the individual patient anatomy, and the length of the remaining right colon and viable transverse colon. Sometimes, division of the middle colic bundle will make a portion of the distal colon ischemic and that will need to be resected. In these cases, the surgeon should consider using fluorescent technology to assess colon perfusion.

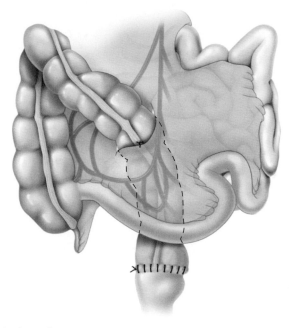

Figure 16-1. Retroileal colorectal anastomosi.

Retroileal colorectal anastomosis (Figure 16-1):

- Divide the middle colic vessels.
- Make sure the blood supply is intact to the transverse colon through the marginal artery.
- A window is created in the mesentery of the ileum. It is important to transilluminate the ileum mesentery to accomplish this safely.
- The distal transverse colon is brought through that defect to enable colorectal anastomosis.
- A downside of this technique is internal herniation and small bowel obstruction.

Deloyer's procedure can be done to reestablish gastrointestinal continuity:

- The hepatic flexure, the ascending colon, and cecum should be completely mobilized.
- Division of the middle colic vessels should be done.
- The ileocolic pedicle should be preserved to supply the cecum and the ascending colon.
- An appendectomy should be performed.
- The cecum is turned 180° anticlockwise around the axis of the ileocolic vessel (Figure 16-2).
- The hepatic flexure by now should be reaching the pelvis. The anastomosis should be between the hepatic flexure and the rectum.

If despite the above maneuvers, making a connection safely seems impossible, then the surgeon has the following options:

1. To fashion an end colostomy and leave the rectal stump. This option leaves the possibility of attempting reconnection open and should be chosen if the discussion about a permanent ostomy or total colectomy or proctocolectomy has not been had with the patient. It is also

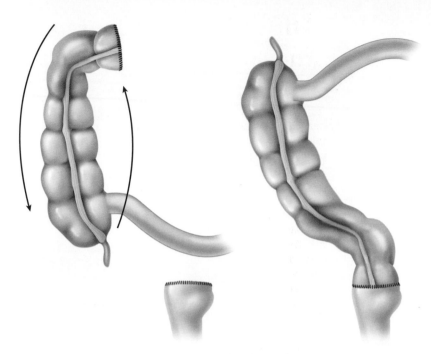

Figure 16-2. Direction of rotation of right colon in Deloyer's procedure.

important if the factors leading to inability of making a connection are considered reversible, i.e., morbid obesity or surgical expertise . This is also a good option for patients who are not a good candidate for an ileostomy or ileorectal anastomosis/ileal pouch anal anastomosis (IPAA) (e.g., baseline sphincter dysfunction/baseline renal dysfunction).

2. Completion colectomy with ileorectal anastomosis (IRA). This option restores intestinal continuity at the expense of resection of the remaining colon. These patients will need to have excellent sphincter function so that they can have good long-term functional outcomes.

3. Completion proctocolectomy with IPAA. This option restores intestinal continuity at the expense of resection of the remaining colon and rectum. This option would only be chosen if the original pathology made a total or near total proctectomy necessary, otherwise an IRA is preferrable. These patients will need to have excellent sphincter function so that they can have good long-term functional outcomes.

4. Completion colectomy with end ileostomy. Here, the rectal stump can be left in situ as a Hartmann's pouch. This would be chosen in patients who have sphincter dysfunction and thus are not a good candidate for IRA or IPAA. This would also be appropriate for patients who are not good candidates for IPAA and have short rectal stumps, making them a poor candidate for an IRA.

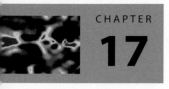

Difficulties with Extracting the Specimen

Difficulties with extracting the specimen are a frequent problem; however, they can be avoided by proper planning. It is important to make sure that adequate mobilization has been carried out intracorporeally before attempting to extract the specimen. The incision has to be tailored to the size of the specimen. The maximum transverse dimension of a tumor in cancer cases should be known to the operating surgeon and the extraction incision should be at least of that size to avoid fracturing of the specimen during extraction. Similarly, when extracting proctectomy specimens, the surgeon has to make allowance for a bulky mesorectum and make the extraction incision accordingly. If there is a struggle in extracting the mesorectum, it may tear leading to a suboptimal specimen. Prior to extraction, one has to make sure that the specimen is mobilized and completely free from the surrounding structures. It helps to place the specimen back in its anatomical position and utilized gravity to make sure the small intestine is not entangled in a way which will make extraction difficult. The exact patient positioning that will facilitate smooth specimen extraction will depend on whether it is a right colon resection, left colon resection, or low anterior resection that is being carried out. It is best to make a longer mark on the skin with a marking pen at the proposed extraction site so that if the incision has to be enlarged it remains in a straight line. We routinely use a wound protector during extraction of the specimens. If facing difficulty during extraction, the following factors should be looked into:

- Sometimes, there will be a suction effect created inside the abdominal cavity during attempts at extraction. Insert your index finger and sweep around the colon to break that suction effect. This will also make sure that a portion of the specimen is not entrapped under the wound protector.

- Make sure that the incision is big enough. Place your index finger while you are pulling and assess if that difficulty is due to a small incision. Sometimes, it helps to extract the appendices epiploicae using the index finger as they may be the reason why the specimen is stuck in a snug incision. If that does not help, extend the incision cranially or caudally and retry.

- If the colon was not returned back to its normal anatomical position prior to extraction, it can get intertwined with small intestine loops, causing difficulty in extraction. This should not happen but is something to be kept in mind, especially if you come in to help someone else during the extraction phase of the operation. If not sure then insufflate and take a look laparoscopically.

- Difficulty in extraction could be because of unrecognized attachments/incomplete mobilization. When the colon is exteriorized and pulled, an index finger is inserted, and these attachments can be felt and divided.

- If it is not easy to divide these or specimen extraction is unusually difficult for any reason then re-insufflate the abdomen and reassess.

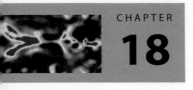

Management of Intraoperative Bleeding Complications During Laparoscopic Colectomy

Major bleeding is one of the most frightening events that can happen to a surgeon in the operating room (OR), especially in minimally invasive procedures. Having a system in mind to approach the problem is essential to help tackle the issue in an organized way.

In all cases of bleeding, follow the algorithm (Figure 18-1).

The Bleeding Inferior Mesenteric Artery

- Division of the inferior mesenteric artery (IMA) is an essential step in all left colon and rectal operations, especially in oncological resections.

- High ligation of the IMA is defined as division of the vessel proximal to the left colic artery takeoff, and low ligation when the IMA is divided after the left colic artery takeoff.

- Division of the IMA can be achieved by different ways. The IMA can be controlled by vessel sealing device (such as LigaSure), bipolar, clips, Endoloop a stapler, or combination of different methods.

- Injury to the IMA a major intraoperative complication that might happen during the division of the vessel and swift action is needed.

Reasons That Could Lead to IMA Injury

Heavily Calcified IMA

This can be seen from the preoperative computed tomography (CT) scan. Occasionally, the energy device will not be able to control the vessel completely, and thus leads to bleeding when the vessel is divided. If the patient is known to have significant atherosclerosis, and there was calcification on preoperative CT scan, then consider using clips or staples rather than an energy source to control the vessel, or modify the technique and use clips in the proximal side of the IMA "staying side" and then using an energy source distally or use Endoloop on the proximal stump in addition to the energy device.

Excessive Tension

If the surgeon and assistant are focusing completely on the IMA dissection, and are not paying attention to the amount of tension that is exerted to lift up the mesentery of the sigmoid

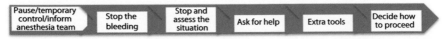

Figure 18-1. Algorithm to deal with any major bleeding.

colon upward, then excessive traction can lead to injury to the IMA especially after the dissection around the IMA is started or during the division of the IMA. This can be avoided if the assistant and the surgeon who is pulling the mesentery upward relax completely during division of the IMA.

Failure of the Instruments

Although failure of the energy device is rare, if it happens, it can lead to a major intraoperative bleeding.

Injury to the IMA While Skeletonizing the Vessel

"Over skeletonizing" the IMA might lead to an injury. An example is by using the laparoscopic scissors to skeletonize the IMA, and injury happens from the back blade of the scissors.

Steps to Control Bleeding

If bleeding is encountered during the division of the IMA, consider following these steps.

First Step: Temporarily Control the Bleeding

- If the bleeding is coming from a side injury to the IMA, then grasping the IMA at the site of injury using an atraumatic grasper can control the bleeding temporarily. Immediately inform the anesthesia team that there may be rapid blood loss.

- If the bleeding is coming from a divided IMA that has a long stump, then use an atraumatic grasper to hold the stump of the IMA. Attempt to do that in a timely fashion, otherwise, pooling of the blood will prevent you from doing so. Use laparoscopic suction as well to help you to identify the vessel before holding it. **NEVER** do anything blindly. It never works, and in fact, you might cause more injury. If you were able to hold the vessel, make sure not to pull it while holding the vessel, because it might injure the vessel even further, and can convert a temporary controlled situation to catastrophic uncontrollable bleeding. If you achieve this, go to the Second Step.

- If the bleeding is coming from a divided IMA that has a short stump, then most likely it will be very difficult to grasp it. At that point, apply pressure with the atraumatic grasper. This will not control the bleeding completely, but it might at least decrease the rate of the bleeding. You have to make the decision **NOW** if you will convert to open or attempt to control it laparoscopically. If decided to attempt to control it laparoscopically, then place a Ray-Tec sponge inside the abdomen, and place it on the bleeding vessel and apply pressure. This move will require you to upsize one of the 5-mm ports, or add an extra port. I would not recommend removing the camera and place the Ray-Tec sponge through it to avoid losing sight on the bleeding vessels, unless you have the vessel under complete control.

If you have achieved control, excellent work. Now go to the Second Step.

- If the bleeding is coming from a stump that is short and can't be grasped, then apply pressure as soon as possible with a Ray-Tec sponge or directly using the atraumatic grasper, and convert to open right away, and don't waste valuable time. Skip the Second Step and go to the Third Step.

Second Step: Stop Completely and Assess the Situation

- Take a deep breath. Assess the situation. Assess how much blood was lost.
- Decide how you will manage this problem now. Still think about converting to open if in doubt. Be a SAFE surgeon. The aim is to get the patient out of the OR with minimum complications.

- Do not rush to do anything "quickly" to fix the problem. If you did not give yourself time to think about it and follow the steps, you will make errors. The patient has already lost blood, your team is not ready, and you may not have the appropriate instruments.

Third Step: Get the Team with You

- Communicate with the anesthesia team about the possibility of major bleeding, so they can request blood from the blood bank, or, if appropriate, activate the massive transfusion protocol.
- Alert the nursing team so everyone is focused.
- Ask for an extra circulating nurse to be in the room so that the nurse can help bring the instruments that were not planned for, while keeping the circulating nurse to help out in the OR.

Fourth Step: Ask for Help

Ask for extra help early from a senior staff, if possible. Another surgeon can be of great help, since they will not be under the same amount of stress as the primary surgeon. If a vascular surgeon is available, this will be a plus.

Fifth Step: Extra Tools

Request the following items to be in the OR, to be ready if needed:

- A headlight in case you convert to open. This will provide better visualization.
- An extra suction unit. This will help significantly at the time of definitive repair because it will provide a clear field while you are repairing the injured vessel.
- A laparotomy tray to be ready in case the decision is made to convert to open.
- A vascular tray.
- Laparoscopic needle holders/vessel loops/clips/additional hemostatic devices (vascular stapler, etc.).

Sixth Step: Make a Decision and Tackle the Problem

- Make the decision on if you will convert to open to control the vessel or attempt to control the vessel laparoscopically.
- Make sure the person who is holding the camera keeps a "safe" distance away from the bleeding to prevent staining the camera with blood. This might lead to losing the window to control the bleeding.
- Options to use to control the bleeding vessel:
  - Energy device
  - Clips
  - Stapler
  - Laparoscopic suturing
  - Endoloop (Figures 18-2 and 18-3)
- Always think ahead and ask for other instruments to be in the room, in case the first method to control the bleeding did not work.
- If the bleeding is temporarily controlled with a grasper, consider dissecting the IMA more proximally to lengthen the IMA stump, if possible and safe, and then control it with a clip.
- Always consider adding extra ports if the plan to control the bleeding laparoscopically.

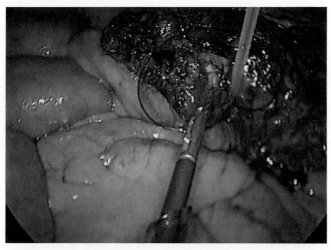

Figure 18-2. Controlling the IMA pedicle using a laparoscopic grasper, and applying the Endoloop to control the pedicle after failure of the energy source.

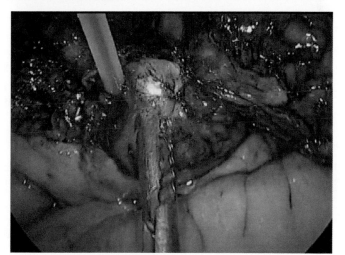

Figure 18-3. Securing the Endoloop to control the IMA.

- There are several methods to control major hemorrhage. The surgeon must use the method that they are most experience with. One trick if you are going to control venous bleeding by laparoscopic suturing is to place a clip at the end of the suture prior to starting the suturing. When the suturing is done, the suture is pulled gently, and another clip is applied. (https://www.sages.org/video/v026-techniques-for-laparoscopic-repair-of-major-intra-operative-vascular-injury/)

Points to Consider During Controlling the IMA

- If the vessel is heavily calcified, consider using two methods to control the IMA. Keep in mind that an energy source alone might not be enough.
- At that point prior to dividing the IMA, make sure that there is an atraumatic grasper very close to the staying side of the stump in case that there will be bleeding. By doing this extra cautious step it will help the surgeon to control the stump right away and prevent massive bleeding.

- Avoid "over skeletonizing" the IMA.
- Avoid excessive pulling of the mesentery of the sigmoid colon and relax while dividing the vessel.

The Bleeding Middle Colic Vessels

If you did not take the middle colic vessels intracorporeally, this will tether the colon during extraction. If you did not take it intracorporeally, be mindful that if you apply excessive traction, this will tear and cause MAJOR bleeding. You will see the evidence of this careless move very quickly when you see gushes of blood from the wound. If this happens, you should consider the following:

First Step: Stop the Bleeding or Temporarily Control the Bleeding

- To do that, the incision has to be extended cranially in a timely fashion (i.e., convert to open). Inform the anesthesia team that there is major ongoing bleeding.
- Pack, pack, and pack. This is the opposite of a trauma case where the site of the bleeding upon entry to the abdomen is not clear and each quadrant has to be packed; you know where the bleeding is coming from. Remove the clots and pack right away in the upper abdomen. If you are able to stop it, hold pressure, take a deep breath, and then go to the next step.

Second Step: Stop Completely and Assess the Situation

- Take a deep breath. Assess the situation. Assess the blood loss. Check if you need to extend the incision even further for adequate exposure in preparation to repair the injury.
- Do not rush to do anything "quickly" to fix the problem. If you do not give yourself time to think about it and follow the steps, you will make errors. The patient has already lost blood, your team is not ready, and you may not have the appropriate instruments.

Third Step: Get the Team with You

- Inform the anesthesia team about the exact situation including the amount of blood loss and whether you have control, so they can request blood from the blood bank, or, if appropriate, activates the massive transfusion protocol.
- Alert the nursing team so everyone is focused and ready to provide help.
- Ask for an extra circulating nurse to be in the room so that the nurse can help bring instruments that were not planned for, while keeping the circulating nurse to help out in the OR.

Fourth Step: Ask for Help

Ask for extra help early from a senior staff, if possible. A senior general or colorectal surgeon can be of great help, since they will not be under the same amount of stress as the primary surgeon. If a vascular surgeon is available, this will be a plus.

Fifth Step: Extra Tools

Request the following items to be in the OR, to be ready if needed:

- A headlight. This will provide better visualization.
- An extra suction unit. This will help significantly at the time of definitive repair, because it will provide a clear field while you are repairing the injured vessel.
- A vascular tray.

- A Bookwalter retractor or any kind or self-retaining retraction for optimal exposure.
- Ask the scrub nurse to prepare multiple 2-0 and 3-0 Prolene sutures already mounted on a long needle driver and ready to use.
- When you use the pool sucker, remove the outer sheath and use the inside part because it's thin, and it will not block your visualization.

Sixth Step: Make a Decision and Tackle the Problem

- Control the bleeding using multiple 2-0 or 3-0 Prolene sutures in a figure of eight fashion.
- After the suture is tied, leave a long tail, so you can reevaluate the area again and it will lead you directly to the bleeding vessel, because after you tie it, it will retract, and if the vessel is not controlled, it will continue to bleed, but the exposure will be more difficult.

Bleeding from the Trocar Site

Bleeding from the trocar site can be either superficial, from the skin or subcutaneous tissue, or it could be from injuring a vessel during inserting the trocar such as the inferior epigastric vessels. If the bleeding was superficial, simple cauterization can be enough to control it.

If the bleeding is coming from the inferior epigastric vessels, then at that point, consider doing any of the following:

- Apply pressure directly using the same trocar, by pushing the trocar against the abdominal wall. This will push the end of the trocar, which is inside the abdomen, toward the abdominal wall from inside and it will apply pressure on the bleeding site.
- Insert a Foley catheter through the trocar, and then inflate the balloon and pull it up against the abdominal wall firmly after the trocar is pulled out, to stop the bleeding, and then hemostat can be placed on the Foley, which is at the level of the skin so this will keep.
- Use a vessel-sealing device (LigaSure) or Bipolar to directly coagulate the bleeding vessel using another port.
- Alternatively, a suture passer can be used to pass a suture around the bleeding vessel and can be tied to control the bleeding

To avoid the inferior epigastric vessels:

- Prior to inserting the trocar, visualize the abdominal wall using the laparoscopic camera, and check for the vessels in the abdominal wall from the inside the abdomen prior to inserting the trocar. In thin patients, transillumination will help to identify the vessel.
- Insert the trocar lateral to the rectus muscle.
- The angle of insertion of the trocar should be 90° perpendicular to the skin.
- Be aware that the course of the inferior epigastric vessel is variable, and the left inferior epigastric vessel is closer to the midline than the right inferior epigastric vessel. However, as a general rule, inferior epigastric vessels are usually located in the area between 4 and 8 cm from the midline.

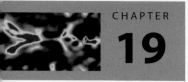

Misadventure with Stapling Devices

The Bad Move: Going Through the Staple Line in the Rectal Stump

One of the most devastating intraoperative complications from circular stapler use is going through the rectal stump. This occurs when the operator loses control while inserting the circular stapler and goes through the transverse staple line. This is most likely to happen when the rectal stump is very short. Usually during insertion of the circular stapler, there is a "give" just as the operator traverses the sphincter muscles. If one is not careful to introduce the stapler in a controlled fashion through the sphincters, they can tear right through the transverse staple line in the lower rectum.

Obviously at that point in surgery, the surgical team is tired and exhausted. Take a deep breath, and keep in mind that it will take patience and time to fix the problem.

In case there is enough length of the rectal stump:

- Dissect the rectal stump circumferentially, and then staple again below that area.

- If that is not an option due to any reason, then perform a purse string suture around the spike of the circular stapler. If you are not able to sew laparoscopically, then convert to open to do this.

If the rectal stump is very short:

- Handsewn coloanal anastomosis can be done.

- Place a purse string on the rectal stump—either laparoscopically or open—and pass the pin of the circular stapler through it and then tie the purse string snug onto it. This is quite challenging in morbidly obese and in male patients. Robotic surgery facilitates this step as sewing is easier. If technically not feasible, then one can do a handsewn anastomosis.

- If adequate length of the proximal colon is available, then one can perform the Turnbull-Cutait procedure (Figure 19-1) where the colon is pulled through the anal canal without anastomosis as a first stage. It followed later by a second operation, and handsewn coloanal anastomosis is performed.

Salvage options if performing an anastomosis is deemed technically impossible:

- Leave the stump open, place an omental pedicle on it, and place a rectal drain and pelvic drain with end colostomy.

- Convert the operation to an intersphincteric abdominoperineal resection (APR). In most cases where ultralow rectal anastomosis is anticipated, the patient should have been counseled for possibility of an intersphincteric APR. However, if that is not the case, then the surgeon should scrub out and talk to the family before proceeding. If they are not in agreement to proceed with an intersphincteric proctectomy then the option described above (end colostomy + drains) should be used.

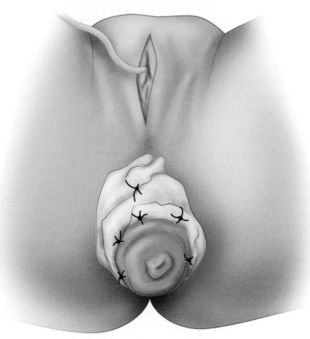

Figure 19-1. Immediate post operative appearance after a Tunbull-Cutait procedure. (Reproduced with permission from Dr. Sherief Shawki.)

The Circular Stapler That Won't Come Out

Sometimes, the circular EEA stapler gets "stuck" after it is fired and does not come out as per routine. In this scenario, several possibilities should be considered.

- This could purely be a device failure.
- This could be an operator error if the person does not know how to correctly use the stapler. Although this is unlikely, it must be ruled out when working with an inexperienced assistant. Different manufactures have guidelines regarding how the stapler should be withdrawn. The operator should be conversant with the type of stapler and the steps that need to be followed for appropriate withdrawal.
- This could be related to inappropriate firing of the device. Folding over of the rectal stump can occur if the rectal stump is not fully effaced by the stapler before the spike is advanced. This can lead to a valve like effect preventing smooth withdrawal of the stapler. Thus, it is important to use appropriately sized stapler based on the patient's anatomy and on the thickness of the rectum. Effacing the rectal stump with the circular stapler prior to advancing the spike is the correct technique and may prevent this problem.

Once this scenario is encountered, follow these steps:

- Take a deep breath and stay calm.
- Make sure that the dial is turned on the stapler for four half turns, which should be done after the EEA stapler is fired (this is manufacturer dependent so follow the guidelines of the device

you are using). This will turn the anvil sideways to facilitate the removal of the instrument. If that is done, and the stapler is still stuck, then continue opening the dial to open the stapler completely.

● If, despite opening the stapler and gentle traction, the stapler does not come out, then it is held in place and the next course of action depends on how high the anastomosis is. If it is within 10 cm from the anal verge, it may be accessible with a digital rectal examination. A gentle rectal examination on the side of the stapler may reveal a cause such as a portion of undivided tissue stuck onto the stapler. If it is high, then you may have to use flexible sigmoidoscopy for visualization of the problem. Flexible sigmoidoscopy can be used even for the low anastomosis. If a lot of tissue is stuck onto the stapler or very thick tissue is stuck raising concern of causing anastomotic disruption while attempting to remove the stapler, then one should strongly consider redoing the entire anastomosis. The stapler may have to be released by dividing the tissue with the help of a laparoscopic scissors passed transanally and by the side of the stapler. If the anastomosis is high, you can divide the anastomosis laparoscopically to release the stapler and redo the entire anastomosis. It is prudent not to forcefully pull out the stapler even when considering redoing the entire anastomosis as it may cause a longitudinal tear of the rectal stump beyond the level of the anastomosis. If the scenario seems salvageable, then try these maneuvers:

○ Try to move the stapler gently in arc shape and gently pull it out. If there is significant resistance, then stop. Many times, the stapler will come out without the anvil. One can use a flexible sigmoidoscopy to assess why the anvil got caught. Most often, it's due to a bridge of extra tissue that was not divided by the stapler. At that point, under direct visualization, use an endoscopic knife to divide that tissue which is holding the anvil using flexible sigmoidoscopy. An endoscopic biopsy forceps can be used to hold the anvil and drag it out. If that does not work, then a snare may be used. For mid to low anastomoses, Ballenger sponge forceps (ring forceps) (Figure 19-2) should be lubricated and inserted and under direct vision of the flexible sigmoidoscope or using a finger in case of low anastomosis, hold the anvil and retrieve it.

○ Alternative to the biopsy forceps, one can use laparoscopic scissors to divide that extra tissue that is holding the anvil under endoscopic guidance.

● After that, flexible sigmoidoscopy is done again to check the anastomosis and make sure there is no defect. In addition, a leak test is performed.

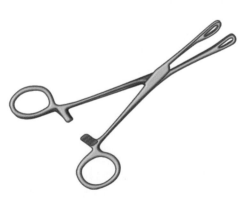

Figure 19-2. Ring forceps.

Difficulties with Inserting the Stapler into the Anus/Rectal Stump

- Sometimes, difficulties inserting the circular stapler are encountered. Make sure to use generous lubrication during digital rectal examination.

- Digitalize the anus with one finger, and then gradually up to 2–3 fingers if the anus feels tight.

- Use the different three sizes of the sizers and insert them into the anal canal. Keep the head of the sizer around the anus to help dilate it. When doing this, be very careful not to push through the rectal stump in case of a low rectal staple line.

- Consider using the size-28 circular stapler rather than 31/33.

- While you are attempting to insert the stapler, make sure to do it in a controlled fashion, to avoid going through the staple line of the rectal stump.

- Occasionally, if the above is not helpful, keep two fingers in the anus, while placing the circular stapler while you lower your hand holding the stapler to insert it at an angle. Try to introduce part of the circular stapler, and then lift up your hand to the neutral position and complete inserting the stapler, while you remove your finger(s) (like using a shoe horn).

The Circular Stapler Won't Reach the End of the Rectal Stump

Occasionally, there will be difficulties with inserting the circular stapler to the end of the rectal stump. This could be due to:

1. Narrow rectum/rectosigmoid from disuse or scarring.
2. Acute angulation in the rectosigmoid area.
3. Scarring from prior disease/surgery with inadequate rectal mobilization.
4. Presence of inspissated stool/mucus especially if the patient had a prior Hartman procedure.

When this is encountered, it is ideal for the more experienced surgeon to make sure that the difficulty is not a manifestation of technical trouble in the hands of a less experienced operator. One must make sure that the end of the operating table is not hindering the manipulation of the circular stapler as well. Also, ensure that adequate lubrication is being used on the circular stapler head.

- After a proper rectal exam (which will demonstrate presence of stool, etc.), use the smallest sizer (25 Fr) with ample lubricant and introduce it to the end of the rectal stump. Assess the angulation and the orientation of the sizer. Place then the medium and large sizers and do the same maneuver, then insert the stapler again. Sometimes, a web or just straightening the rectum with the sizer could solve this issue.

- If the sizer can't reach the end, then one has to assess the reason for this. If the operator is hubbed at the anus (i.e., there is no length left on the stapler handle to be inserted further), then the end of the rectosigmoid stump may be too high and may need resection. It is best to mark the level of resection by scoring the mesocolon/mesorectum or marking an appendicis epiploica with cautery, this should be done with the circular stapler in situ and resect the extra rectosigmoid. There may be severe angulation preventing the stapler from advancing. Consider further mobilization of the rectum and try again. If this fails, re-resect the rectal stump to an area where the stapler can reach. Also, consider using a smaller size stapler 28–29 mm if the 31–33 mm stapler was used initially. However, this will require removal of the anvil and revision of the purse string suture proximally.

- If inspissated stool or mucus plug is the cause, then it can be manually removed while the surgeon "milks" it down using a laparoscopic bowel grasper or removes it via flexible sigmoidoscopy.

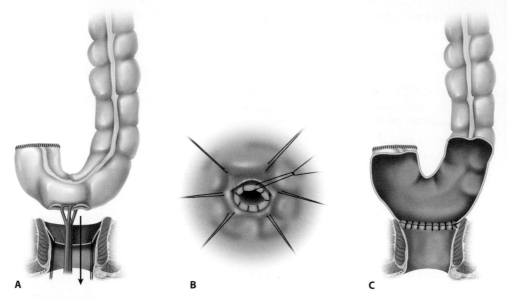

Figure 19-3. End-to-side anastomosis.

To avoid this, fleet enema should be given preoperatively, especially if the planned operation is Hartman's reversal where the rectal stump can contain inspissated mucus and stool.

- Alternatively, introduce the spike where the stapler can maximally reach on the anterior wall of the rectum, to create an end-to-side anastomosis (Figure 19-3). However, there must be a few centimeters distance between the circular stapler line and the TA staple line in the rectum, otherwise, the tissue in between may become ischemic and lead to a leak.

Failure of the Liner Stapler During Vascular Ligation/Nuances of Vascular Ligation Using an Energy Device

One of the methods to control the inferior mesenteric artery (IMA) or the ileocolic pedicle is using the linear stapler. If this staple line fails, massive bleeding will happen that might require blood transfusion, and conversion to open surgery.

One of the ways to address this issue is to anticipate that this could happen and prevent it. Here are few tips:

- Make sure there is enough length of the vessel dissected before ligation. If the vessel is not dissected and cleared enough, it will be difficult to identify and control it if the staple line fails.
- Before proceeding, make sure that the Endoloop ligature is available in the OR, in case there is failure of the staple line.
- When the vessel is ligated, make sure not to divide the vessel flush with the aorta. Make sure there is enough space proximal to the area of ligation "stump" that it can be grabbed if the staple line fails (a 1-cm stump should suffice). If the division is made as close to the origin of the vessel as possible, if there is a problem with the stapler, or whatever method is used, it will lead to a hole in the aorta which will be very difficult to manage. Such a scenario would likely need conversion to open with direct suture repair of the aorta in order to control the bleeding.

- The assistant should not put excessive traction on the mesentery while retracting the vascular pedicle prior to, and during ligation. This is especially important when part of the artery is divided with a sealing device or stapler and the rest of it may avulse if excessive traction is used for retraction.

- If an energy source is used, three points of ligation are used. The vessel is sealed proximally first, 0.5–1 cm distal to the origin. Then the vessel is sealed distally, and then finally, sealed in between the two areas and divided. Make sure there is overlap in the area of the vessel that is sealed (Figure 19-4). When the vessel is divided using an energy source, make sure to use the cutting mechanism halfway, meaning that the vessel should not be divided all the way after sealing it the first time. It is partially divided. Then, apply the energy source again to the remaining part, and then divide the vessel completely (Figure 19-5). This is done by partially squeezing the trigger.

- During division of the vessel, the nondominant hand of the operator or the assistant should have a Maryland grasper close to the "stump" of the vessel, just in case there is a failure of the energy source or the stapler, and the stump can be grabbed as quickly as possible with the grasper. In that case, the vessel will be under control quickly with minimal bleeding. Either Endoloop ligature or laparoscopic clips can be used to control the vessel, or the energy source can be used. (It's a good idea to avoid using the same technique of controlling the vessel, if it failed initially.)

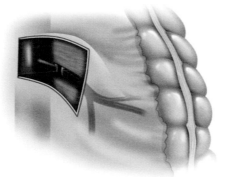

Figure 19-4. Depiction of the "double burning" of a blood vessel just before division using a vessel sealing device.

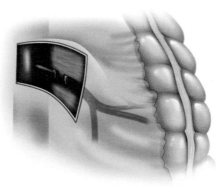

Figure 19-5. Blood vessel divided after "double burning" with a larger portion of the sealed vessel on the "staying" side and a smaller portion on the specimen side.

How to Avoid Errors and Misadventures of the Circular Stapler

Following a good technique and sound judgment during the bowel preparation for the anastomosis and during constructing the anastomosis is paramount to decrease the incidence of avoidable errors using the circular stapler.

Here are few points to keep in mind:

- Make sure that the patient is low enough on the OR table to prevent any obstacles when the stapler is moved to any direction.
- Make sure the bowel used for anastomosis is not chronically dilated or hypertrophied, otherwise, the tissue may be too thick for a stapled anastomosis.
- While preparing the proximal colon, and after creating the purse string suture, make sure to clear the fat and extra-tissue around the anvil where it will be joined with the stapler to make the anastomosis.
- While creating the purse string suture, use a monofilament suture, usually a 2-0 Prolene suture, to prevent "bunching up," which can lead to incomplete apposition caused by leaving part of the bowel edges lying outside the anvil.
- Likewise, when the stapler is inserted in the rectal stump, make sure the stapler is fully effaced prior to introducing the spike. After the spike is introduced, do not withdraw the stapler and keep it effaced.
- The operator can place an open jaw of the atraumatic grasper over the stamp to help the spike to go through the rectal stump.
- Effective and clear communication between the operator and the first assistant who is inserting the stapler in the anal canal is paramount to avoid any errors. It is worth reviewing the steps of stapling with the first assistant if they are a trainee. The operator should guide the assistant with the direction of the stapler very clearly.
- During stapling, the assistant should remove the safety and use both hands to fire the stapler. Uncontrolled movements during that time could lead to misfiring. It is best to lower the level of the bed so it is easier to fire the stapler.
- After the stapler is fired, the assistant should keep holding for 15–20 seconds before release.
- After the stapler is released, the safety should be returned. The stapler is opened by four half turns, and this puts the anvil at the ideal angle for removal.
- Very gently, the assistant should start moving the stapler in an arc movement and remove the stapler, while keeping in mind to look at the laparoscopy screen where it's showing the anastomosis.
- We routinely perform flexible sigmoidoscopy after creating the anastomosis. There are a few advantages of performing flexible sigmoidoscopy after constructing the anastomosis:
  - Visualize the anastomosis and make sure it's intact without any defect.
  - Make sure the hemostasis is adequate. Most of the bleeding that occurs from the staple line is self-limited; however, if there is massive bleeding or an obvious spurting vessel, an endoscopic clip can be applied.
  - Assess the bowel just proximal to the anastomosis and make sure the color of the bowel is normal, and there is no evidence of ischemia. No need to go past the scope through the anastomosis.
  - Perform the leak test:
    1. Decrease the degree of the Trendelenburg position a little so that the irrigation stays in the pelvis.

2. Immerse the anastomosis with saline or water.

3. Gently place an atraumatic grasper on the proximal bowel to occlude it completely to test the anastomosis.

4. Insufflation of the neo-rectum is performed just proximal to the anastomosis.

5. Make sure not to insufflate excessively.

- In case of positive leak test, follow the steps in Figure 19-6.

The four critical things to make sure before constructing any anastomosis are:

- There should be no twist in the mesocolon. Follow the cut edge of the mesentery of the left colon, and follow that until the splenic flexure.

- Make sure that the anastomosis is under no tension whatsoever. The cost of this will be dire. Make sure that the left colon and the splenic flexure are completely mobilized. The left colon should lie in the pelvis with slight slack and should not be on a stretch when it is brought down to the level of the proposed anastomosis.

- Make sure there is no small bowel under the colon, where it could lead to postoperative bowel obstruction due to internal hernia (i.e., there should not be small bowel to the left of the colon).

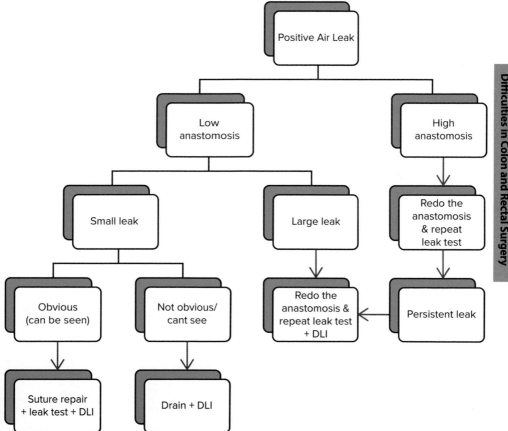

Figure 19-6. Diverting loop ileostomy (DLI).

- Adequate blood supply:

  ○ The Pinpoint Endoscopic Fluorescence Imaging System: After using a bolus of indocyanine green (ICG), the proximal, distal colon and the anastomosis (after it gets constructed) are checked using a special camera and light source optimized for high-definition white light and near infrared fluorescence images. This will allow to detect if there is any compromise in the blood supply of the bowel.

  ○ Alternatively, while preparing the proximal end of the left colon and prior to inserting the anvil, divide the appendices epiploica or fat and look for bleeding. If there is bleeding, then most likely the blood supply is adequate. If not, revise the margin and use more proximal bowel.

How to Avoid Incorporating the Vagina During the Stapling

In female patients, additional steps should be followed to make sure that the vagina is not incorporated in the stapler. The development of a colovaginal fistula is a preventable complication, and great care should be exercised prior to firing the circular stapler to avoid this complication.

In mid-to-low rectal anastomosis, make sure of the following:

- During the anterior dissection of the rectum, the vagina should be identified and pushed upward. This dissection should be continued to completely push the vagina away from the rectal wall.

- During inserting the circular stapler, make sure it is inserted in the rectum. It might sound so obvious, but this could happen especially in patients with a very high BMI. Insert the left index finger in the vagina, while with your right hand, insert the stapler in the anal canal.

- After the anvil and the spike of the stapler are joined and the stapler is closed, but before firing the stapler, the vagina should be visualized laparoscopically and pulled away from the anastomosis. In very low anastomosis with poor laparoscopic visualization, insert a finger in the vagina, and then very gently move the stapler only few millimeters and check if there is any pulling in the vagina. If there is no movement or tugging in the vagina, then fire the stapler.

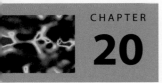

How to Deal with the Difficult Crohn's Mesentery

Division of the mesentery of the bowel is usually an easy step in the operation that can be done without any issue. One of the conditions, which is an exception to the rule, is the mesentery of Crohn's disease. The small bowel mesentery of Crohn's disease will be foreshortened, very thickened, and may be firm/hard. It's not uncommon to encounter bleeding if the usual techniques are used to control the mesentery. Although division of the mesentery can be done laparoscopically or robotically, it will be technically challenging due to risk of bleeding.

There are few techniques to consider:

- Preferably, this part of the procedure is done using open technique after the bowel is exteriorized.

- When exteriorizing the specimen, if the incision is small, have a lower threshold than usual to extend the incision. Pulling on the bowel to exteriorize the thick mesentery may cause tears in the mesentery that causes bleeding.

- One way to get better exposure without extending the incision significantly is to exteriorize the colon, divide it, and place a 3-0 Vicryl suture in the antimesenteric corner and return it back to the abdominal cavity after you tag that suture with hemostat, and then exteriorize the thickened terminal ileum. Sometimes, the mesentery is very thickened and cannot be totally exteriorized via a laparoscopic extraction incision. In this scenario, it may be best to convert to an open operation.

- Using an energy source to divide the mesentery is not recommended because it may not completely seal the mesenteric vessels and will cause bleeding. This is due to the significant thickness and scarring of the mesentery, especially close to the bowel wall. If one uses an energy source then it is best to take the mesentery in layers and further away from the bowel wall where the mesentery may not be as thick as it is close to the bowel wall.

- Score the mesentery superficially.

- Start dividing the mesentery using Kelly clamps and suture ligation to control the mesentery.

- When the mesentery is divided between the Kelly clamps, make sure of the following:
  - Not to divide the mesentery beyond the end of the tip of the Kelly clamp.
  - Divide the mesentery close to the clamp that is on the specimen side, leaving a cuff of tissue on the staying side. Otherwise, the vessel might retract and the tie may slip.

- Multiple small bites of mesentery should be taken when clamping. If one takes large bites then the suture might not control the vessel, because of the thickness of the mesentery (Figure 20-1).

- Use 0 or 2-0 Vicryl to control the mesentery by doing a suture ligature. After you place the first knot, release the Kelly clamp and then re-grab quickly, and complete a

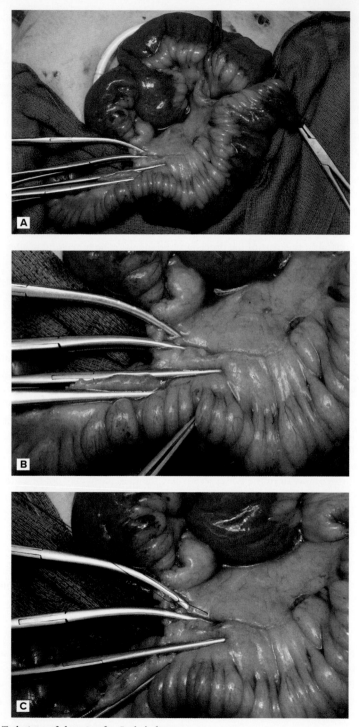

Figure 20-1. Technique of clamping for Crohn's disease.

total of four knots. After that suture is cut, place a free suture and tie it around the Kelly clamp using a sliding knot and make sure it's completely down, but be careful not to tear through the mesentery.

- In case of bleeding, do not panic. Gently hold the mesentery between your fingers using both the thumb and the index fingers. Gentle pressure can control the bleeding until it can be controlled by another suture ligation or free tie. Once you have controlled the bleeder with direct manual pressure, make sure you have two working suctions and Prolene stitches (2-0 or 3-0) on the field. Inform anesthesia to anticipate mild-to-moderate blood loss. Keep them apprised if this changes and when you have definitive control.

- While securing the knot, make sure to push the knot gently to control the vessel, but not carelessly to "rip" through the mesentery.

- If there is still bleeding after the ligation of the mesentery, figure of eight sutures can be used to control the bleeding. It helps to use Prolene sutures in this scenario.

- In laparoscopic cases, make sure to intentionally inspect the mesentery one more time when the laparoscope is reintroduced again at the end of the case to check for bleeding.

Dealing with Complications and Difficulties in Colon and Rectal Surgery

The Morbidly Obese Patient

Surgery in the morbidly obese patient poses unique challenges for the surgeon, compared to those with a normal BMI. Meticulous preoperative planning is imperative in these patients to prevent postoperative complications and allow smooth progression intraoperatively. In this chapter, we will discuss certain technical aspects of minimally invasive colorectal surgery applicable to the obese patient population—a large number of the Western patient population tend to be overweight and, therefore, being able to safely operate on obese patients is essential.

Access

We used the open Hasson technique to access the abdomen in all our cases. However, in the morbidly obese patient, this can be uniquely challenging and time-consuming and so it is reasonable to use a different approach such as the Veress needle or an Optiview. The standard approach with the Veress needle at the Palmer's point may be used followed by an Optiview trocar insertion. In our approach, we still use the open Hasson technique; however, we do so at the point of extraction of the specimen, which allows us to use a larger skin incision to gain access, while keeping the fascial incision small in order to avoid a CO_2 leak during the surgery.

Perioperative Challenges

The morbidly obese patient tends to have comorbidities such as hypertension, diabetes, coronary artery disease, and malnutrition that need to be managed proactively to avoid postoperative surgical morbidities. In patients undergoing surgery for benign conditions or in whom the surgery can be safely deferred for a few weeks to months, it is very beneficial to ask the patient to lose weight, perform prehabilitation in the form of an aerobic exercises, incentive spirometry, physical therapy, smoking cessation if applicable, dietary modification, and weight reduction. Good glucose control and blood pressure control in the perioperative period for those patients with concomitant hypertension and diabetes leads to better outcomes and reduction in surgical morbidity. Postoperative mobilization and ambulation can be a challenge in in the morbidly obese patient and it helps to have early involvement of physical therapist and occupational therapist. Preoperative education about expectations and the need for early mobilization is very helpful in these patients. Lastly, in patients in whom it is deemed appropriate, it may be beneficial to refer the patient to a bariatric surgeon for a bariatric procedure prior to their colorectal surgery or a concomitant bariatric/colorectal operation.

Patient Position and Safety during Surgery

In morbidly obese patients, it is very important to make sure that the patient is properly secured, and the pressure points are padded in order to avoid nerve injuries. This may require use of specialized equipment such as foam or bean bags and the need for additional measures to secure the patient on to the operating room table in the form of additional belts and securing the patient with the help of silk tapes. The need for using extenders in order to secure the arms next to the patient and the need for using foot boards in order to prevent slipping of the patient when they are in an extreme reverse Trendelenburg position should be anticipated and addressed prior to starting the case. It is important for the surgeon to be personally involved during positioning of these patients including the "tilt test" before starting the surgery. During the surgery, it is important to be cognizant for the duration that the patient is in the steep Trendelenburg or reverse Trendelenburg. In our practice, we frequently change the position of the morbidly obese patient in order to avoid position-related injuries and complications. While these risk factors are present in every patient undergoing minimally invasive colorectal surgery, their frequency is enhanced with the additional body weight in morbidly obese patients (see Figure 21-1).

Intraoperative Challenges

Working Space

One of the common challenges noted in morbidly obese patients is the lack of working space despite standard insufflation pressures. This can happen because of a bulky omentum and the body habitus in certain patients who carry most of their adipose tissue intra-abdominally. One can try to create working space by changing the position of the patient and also by using slightly higher insufflation pressures, although we have to be very cognizant of the hemodynamic changes that this may cause and make sure that the anesthesiologist is aware that we are using higher pressures than normal. If, despite higher insufflation pressure and positioning changes, there is not enough working space, the placement of additional trocars may be considered for ease of retraction especially of a bulky omentum to create more space and potentially continue with the operation. If all maneuvers, including the placement of additional ports, do not allow proper visualization and the safe continuation of surgery, then converting to an open operation must be considered early rather than late.

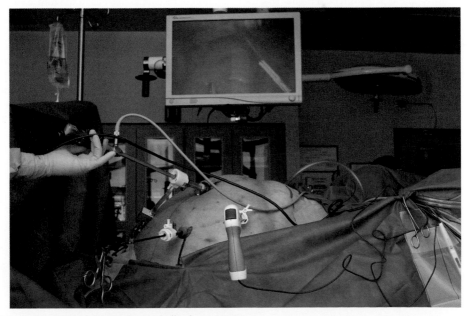

Figure 21-1. Laparoscopy in the morbidly obese patient.

Dealing with Complications and Difficulties in Colon and Rectal Surgery

Identification of the Ureters

In our practice, the threshold for placing ureteric stents in the morbid obese patient population is quite low. It is not uncommon to have difficulty in identifying the ureters in these patients as the retroperitoneum can be quite thick and the usual vermiculation of the ureter may be very difficult to visualize. Of course, the decision to place ureteric stents depends on the pathology and the preoperative imaging findings just like in any other patient, but we favor placing the stents more liberally in the morbidly obese patient.

Thick Mesocolon

The mesocolon tends to be thick in patients with a higher BMI and it may not be safe to divide the mesocolon using an energy device. In this situation, we favor placing Hem-o-lok clips or use the vascular stapler for division of the mesocolon. This decision, of course, is individualized depending on the thickness of the mesocolon and anatomy of the vasculature. It is also dependent on the age of the patient and level of calcification in their blood vessels, which can be evaluated preoperatively on the imaging.

Ostomy Creation/Specimen Extraction

Due to the thick adipose layer in the abdominal wall, both ostomy creation and specimen extraction pose unique challenges for the surgeon in the morbidly obese patient. As a general rule, the abdominal wall tends to be thinner above the level of the umbilicus and it is a good idea to ask the ostomy nurses to mark an option for bringing up the stoma above the level of the umbilicus. Placement of a wound protector device helps in bringing an ostomy up and also helps in specimen extraction to keep the incision small. Sometimes, bringing up an end ileostomy or an end colostomy is not possible because of tethering of the bowel secondary to thick mesentery. In these situations, modification of technique in the form of a loop end colostomy or loop end ileostomy may be needed. Removal of subcutaneous adipose tissue can sometimes help in reduction of the distance needed to bring out the ostomy. These patients have a higher risk for formation of incisional hernias in the future and an off-midline extraction site is preferable; however, this poses a unique challenge as they tend to have pannus, which makes extraction at the Pfannenstiel location more challenging and off midline extraction also tends to be more challenging because of a thicker abdominal wall. However, if feasible, then midline extraction does prevent the formation of incisional hernias; moreover, it is important to have good visualization for completing a closure in the proper fashion, even if this means making a larger skin incision to get proper exposure. When performing an end ostomy in morbidly obese patients, consideration should be given to placement of a prophylactic mesh in order to prevent formation of a hernia in the long term.

Introduction to Robotic Surgery

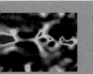

CHAPTER

22

Introduction to Robotic Colorectal Surgery

Robotic surgery has emerged as the third platform that can be used by a colorectal surgeon to perform various resections. Like most new technologies, robotic surgery has had its share of critics and advocates. There are many commercial robotics forms available to colorectal surgeons worldwide. However, the authors' experience is limited to the da Vinci platform and currently, we use the Xi version of the da Vinci robot for most rectal cases including rectopexy and proctectomies. Several surgeons advocate using the robot for all colorectal surgeries including right colectomies. However, in our practice, we still perform the right colectomies laparoscopically partly because it allows us to train the future generation in both laparoscopic and robotic techniques and partly because the biggest advantage of using the robotic platform is in the pelvis where the feet are narrow and further robotic surgery offers certain advantages over both laparoscopic and open surgery in our opinion. For the purpose of this chapter, the robotic platform being discussed will be limited to the da Vinci platform and largely the Xi version.

Advantages of Robotic Surgery

- The surgeon can control three arms. This takes away the dependence on a skilled assistant, especially in a narrow-working field such as the pelvis. This makes the platform more stable as the surgeon controls the camera and two working ports at all times.

- Three-dimensional vision enhances the appreciation of tissue planes and has the potential to minimize injuries to structures such as nerves and blood vessels, especially in the narrow male pelvis.

- The robotic instruments have increased the range of motion even when compared to the human hand. This gives the surgeon the ability to perform complex maneuvers within a very narrow space, allowing precise dissection in the pelvis.

- Ability to switch the field of vision from 30 down to 30 up and vice versa without any physical movement of the camera. The authors have found this feature of the robotic platform to be very helpful during ultra-low dissection of the rectum and rectal transection during proctectomy.
- The robotic platform is ergonomically superior to laparoscopy and open surgery as the surgeon can perform the surgery well seated and does not need to be scrubbed for it.

Disadvantages of the Robotic Platform

- Lack of tactile/haptic feedback. This is an important limitation of the current robotic platform and can potentially lead to tissue injury if the surgeon is not careful and does not follow visual cues in order to adjust the amount of traction being placed on the tissue.
- Narrow field of vision. Compared to the laparoscopic platform, the robotic surgery field of vision tends to be narrower because the camera functions best when it is closer to the operative field. This restricts the "peripheral vision" of the operating surgeon and can lead to unsafe situations especially if the surgeon is not aware of the third arm instrument which may be outside of the operative field.
- Inability to change the patient's position while the robot is docked. This is a disadvantage which can be overcome by procuring a table which can "communicate" with the robot. However, procuring such a table increases the cost of the platform.
- Longer time is required to convert to an open procedure compared to laparoscopy. This advantage becomes apparent if the surgeon wants to emergently convert to an open procedure secondary to bleeding as it takes longer to undock the robot as opposed to laparoscopy. Moreover, the operative surgeon also needs additional time in order to scrub and gown and glove prior to converting to an open surgery.
- Restricted field of surgery. The robotic platform works very well for an operation which has to be conducted in one area of the abdomen such as the pelvis or the gastroesophageal junction but needs to be readjusted if the surgeon wants to operate on a wide field, for example, during total colectomy. The robot may need to be undocked and redocked in order to complete a procedure such as a total colectomy/proctocolectomy.
- Cost has been a major factor which has restricted the use of the robot and has also been one of the main criticisms of this platform. However, over a period of time with more manufacturers building their own robotic platforms and more procedures being performed robotically the cost will likely come down dramatically.

General Principles

The general principles of open and laparoscopic surgery apply to robotic surgery in the sense that the procedure itself remains unchanged; however, the surgeon needs to learn the nuances of the platform and recognize how to utilize its strengths, while reducing the risks secondary to loss of haptic feedback and a narrow field of vision. The following principles should be followed when starting/performing robotic surgery:

- The online modules provided by the manufacture should be completed before a surgeon starts robotic surgery. This is very important to ensure the safe and smooth initiation of a surgeon into the realm of robotic surgery. These modules go over in detail on how to dock and undock the robot and the basic functioning of the robotic console and basics of bedside assisting.
- Before performing the first case it is prudent to practice on the robotic simulator in order to be facile with a platform.
- When the surgeon is ready to dock the robot, they should first dock the robotic camera and perform "targeting" toward the organ that they are operating on, most commonly the rectum

in our practice. Thereafter, each instrument should be brought in under vision after docking all the robotic arms and making sure that there is enough space between each robotic arm and enough clearance between the patient and the robotic arms.

- It is important to be aware of the location of the retracting third arm at all times so that the operating instrument arms do not provide with the third arm which usually is out of the operative field and thus not visible to the surgeon. If the third arm is accidentally moved by the second arm, then the tissue being held by the third arm can be damaged leading to bleeding or spillage of bile or feces.

- It is very important to periodically check the orientation of the camera and the degree of rotation of the camera. This is easily done by looking at the camera icon at the bottom of the screen on the surgical console. Failure to check the orientation of the camera can lead to dissection in the wrong plane or off midline especially in the pelvis.

- Pressure from the robotic arms on the patient can lead to injury and so the bedside assistant has to be very careful about how close the robotic arms get to the patient's body.

Pelvic/Left-Sided Procedures

Si System

- Port placement: see Figures 22-1, 22-2, and 22-3.

Xi System

- The Xi system has made advances which make docking easier and also add flexibility in the positioning of the robotic cart. The system has the ability to rotate at the level of the robotic "boom" thus making it possible to work at all abdominal quadrants with the same port configuration. Performing a total proctocolectomy is feasible with the use of this system without the need for multiple redocking.

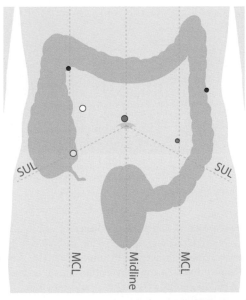

Figure 22-1. Port placement for LAR, Si system. (©2023 Intuitive Surgical Operations, Inc)

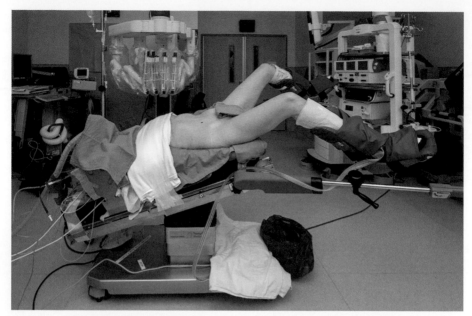

Figure 22-2. Patient positioning for LAR. (Reproduced with permission from El-Ghobashy A, Ind T, Persson J, et al. *Textbook of Gynecologic Robotic Surgery*. Cham, Switzerland: Springer Nature; 2018.)

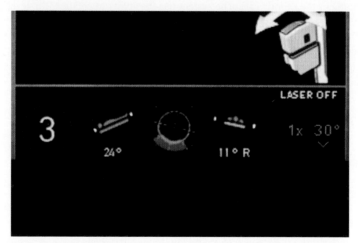

Figure 22-3. Robotic consul demonstrating patient tilt (24 degrees Trendelenburg and 11 degrees "left up") with a 30-degree camera. (Reproduced with permission from El-Ghobashy A, Ind T, Persson J, et al. *Textbook of Gynecologic Robotic Surgery*. Cham, Switzerland: Springer Nature; 2018.)

- Port Placement (see Figure 22-4): four ports are placed in a straight line perpendicular to a line drawn along the axis of the target organ, that is, for an LAR or any pelvic case four ports are placed along a transverse line at the level of the umbilicus. This, however, makes it difficult to use these ports for conventional laparoscopy as they are all in one straight line. The authors' preference is to use a balloon Hasson trocar entry at the assistant port site to obtain pneumoperitoneum and then to use three 8-mm robotic ports and one 12-mm robotic port in the right lower quadrant for stapling.

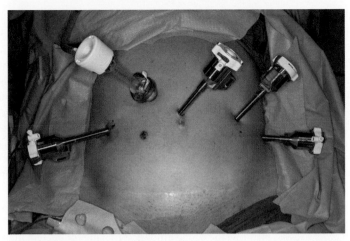

Figure 22-4. Port placement for LAR, Xi system. (Reproduced with permission from El-Ghobashy A, Ind T, Persson J, et al. *Textbook of Gynecologic Robotic Surgery*. Cham, Switzerland: Springer Nature; 2018.)

- Preferred robot docking: over patient's left side.
- Optional robot docking: between legs (this is commonly the position used by the gynecologists).
- Patient positioning: same as Si system above.

Instruments

- Right arm: monopolar scissors/vessel sealing device/robotic stapler
- Left arm: fenestrated bipolar grasper
- Third arm: cardiere
- Midline port: camera (30 degrees)

Assistant

Alternates between suction and bowel grasper.

Key Operative Steps for Low Anterior Resection/Sigmoid Colectomy

1. Abdominal cavity exploration, visualization of entire abdomen including the liver.
2. Exposure of pelvis and sigmoid mesocolon: this is achieved by positioning the patient in steep Trendelenburg (25 degrees or more) and left side up position (10 degrees or more). The small intestine loops are gently retracted out of the pelvis. If there are adhesions, then sharp adhesiolysis is performed. Sometimes a redundant cecum may obscure the view by flopping down into the pelvis and may need to be mobilized and retracted away for exposure of the pelvis. In difficult cases (morbidly obese, multiple prior surgeries, prior radiation, etc.), it helps to introduce a surgical gauze or sterile vaginal packing (cut to desirable length) to help retract the small intestine out of the pelvis.
3. Dissection and ligation of inferior mesenteric artery (IMA) proximal to origin of the superior hemorrhoidal artery. The authors' preference is the vessel-sealing device. Alternatively vascular clips may be used. Ligation of the IMA close to its origin is optimal for maximum length in order to achieve a tension-free anastomosis.
4. Medial to lateral mobilization of sigmoid and left colon.
5. Retro-rectal dissection in the total mesorectal excision plane.

Introduction to Robotic Surgery

6. Rectal division.

7. Splenic flexure mobilization (if indicated). When the splenic flexure needs to be mobilized the authors prefer to divide the inferior mesenteric vein close to the duodena-jejunal flexure. This helps in maximizing the length of the colon and aids in tension-free anastomosis.

8. Specimen extraction. The sites commonly used are the site for diverting loop ileostomy, Pfannenstiel incision, periumbilical incision, and transvaginal extraction. Choice of the site depends on the procedure, the need for extraction of concomitant specimen, bulk of the specimen, patient body habitus, and surgeon preference.

9. Colorectal anastomosis using a circular stapling device. When making the anastomosis, the surgeon must ensure adequate blood supply, proper orientation, and the lack of tension. In addition, the small intestinal loops must be retracted medially so that they are not trapped under the left colon.

10. Loop ileostomy creation (if indicated). It is very important to maintain proper orientation when maturing the loop ileostomy. It is a good practice to mark the afferent and efferent limb in order to avoid maturing the wrong limb (i.e. brooking the efferent limb instead of the afferent limb of the ileal loop). Such an error leads to difficult pouching and excoriation of peristomal skin and the need for revision of the stoma.

Right-Sided Procedures

Si System

- Port placement: see Figure 22-5.

Xi System

- Port placement (see Figure 22-6): four ports are placed in an oblique line drawn along the left of the patient's midline. Port 2 is the camera port.

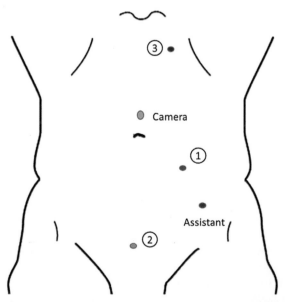

Figure 22-5. Port placement for right colectomy, Si system. (Reproduced with permission from Pappou EP, Weiser MR. Robotic colonic resection. *J Surg Oncol.* 2015;112(3):315-320.)

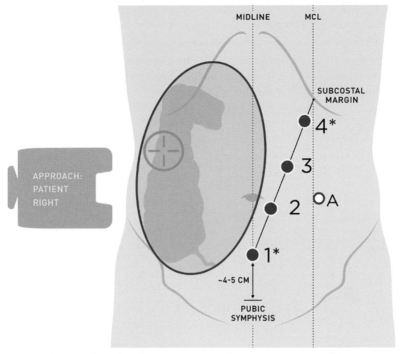

Figure 22-6. Port placement for right colectomy, Xi system. (©2023 Intuitive Surgical Operations, Inc)

- Preferred robot docking: over the patient's right side.
- Patient positioning: same as Si system above.

Instruments

- Right arm: monopolar scissors/vessel sealing device/robotic stapler
- Left arm: fenestrated bipolar grasper
- Third arm: cardiere
- Midline port: camera (30 degrees)

Assistant

Alternates between suction and bowel grasper.

Key Operative Steps for Right Colectomy

1. Abdominal cavity exploration, visualization of entire abdomen including the liver.
2. Exposure of the right colon and ileocolic pedicle: this is done by reflecting the omentum above the transverse colon and the small intestine medially. The cecum is retracted anteriorly and laterally to tent up the ileocolic pedicle.
3. Medial to lateral dissection and delineation of ileocolic pedicle. It is important to prevent trauma to the duodenum.

4. Ileocolic pedicle division and completion of medial to lateral dissection with division of right branch of middle colic artery.

5. Lateral-to-medial dissection with a takedown of hepatic flexure.

6. Anastomosis. This can be extracorporeal or intracorporeal depending on surgeon preference. If an extraction incision is needed for another reason (abdominal hysterectomy, etc.), then there is no inherent advantage of doing an intracorporeal anastomosis.

Index

Note: Page numbers followed by *f* denote figures; by *t*, tables.